CONTENTS

Chapter 1: Introduction to HIV & AIDS 1
Chapter 2: HIV Virology and Biochemistry 14
Chapter 3: Anatomy and Physiology 38
Chapter 4: Clinical Manifestations and Symptoms 58
Chapter 5: Diagnostic Methods 83
Chapter 6: Treatment and Management 99
Chapter 7: Prevention and Public Health Strategies 122
Chapter 8: Societal Impacts and Ethical Considerations 141

CHAPTER 1: INTRODUCTION TO HIV & AIDS

Overview of HIV & AIDS

Human Immunodeficiency Virus (HIV) and Acquired Immunodeficiency Syndrome (AIDS) represent one of the most complex and challenging public health issues of the modern era. HIV, the causative agent of AIDS, primarily targets the immune system, specifically CD4 T-helper cells, leading to progressive immune system failure and susceptibility to opportunistic infections and cancers.

Epidemiology and Global Impact

HIV/AIDS has had a profound impact globally since its recognition in the early 1980s. According to the World Health Organization (WHO), approximately 37.7 million people were living with HIV globally in 2020, with 1.5 million new infections and 680,000 AIDS-related deaths reported. Sub-Saharan Africa remains disproportionately affected, accounting for nearly two-thirds of all people living with HIV worldwide.

Etiology and Transmission

HIV belongs to the retrovirus family and primarily infects CD4 T-cells and macrophages, crucial components of the human immune system. The virus gains entry into these cells through interaction with specific cellular receptors, notably CD4 and either CCR5 or CXCR4 co-receptors. Transmission occurs through exposure to infected bodily fluids, including blood, semen, vaginal fluids, and breast milk, primarily via unprotected sexual intercourse, sharing of contaminated needles, and from mother to child during childbirth or breastfeeding.

Pathogenesis

Upon entry into the host cell, HIV undergoes a complex replication cycle involving reverse transcription of its RNA genome into DNA, integration of viral DNA into the host genome, and subsequent production of new viral particles that mature and are released to infect other cells. HIV's ability to integrate into host DNA and establish latent reservoirs complicates eradication efforts, making lifelong treatment necessary for viral suppression.

Clinical Stages

HIV infection progresses through several clinical stages:

- **Acute HIV Infection:** Initial phase occurring within weeks of exposure, characterized by flu-like symptoms such as fever, rash, sore throat, and swollen lymph nodes. Viral replication is rapid during this stage.
- **Chronic HIV Infection:** Asymptomatic phase where viral replication continues at lower levels, often lasting for several years if untreated.
- **Advanced HIV Infection (AIDS):** Defined by severe immune deficiency, indicated by a CD4 cell count below 200 cells/mm^3 or the occurrence of opportunistic infections and AIDS-defining cancers.

Impact on Immune System

HIV primarily targets CD4 T-helper cells, which play a crucial role in coordinating immune responses. Progressive depletion of CD4 cells weakens the immune system's ability to fight infections and malignancies, leading to the characteristic immunodeficiency seen in AIDS.

Treatment and Prevention

Antiretroviral therapy (ART) represents the cornerstone of HIV treatment, effectively suppressing viral replication and preserving immune function when taken consistently. ART consists of combinations of drugs targeting different stages of the HIV life cycle, including entry inhibitors, reverse transcriptase inhibitors, integrase inhibitors, and protease inhibitors. Prevention strategies include promoting safe sexual practices, needle exchange programs for injecting drug users, pre-exposure prophylaxis (PrEP) for high-risk individuals, and early initiation of ART for people living with HIV to prevent transmission.

Social and Economic Impact

Beyond its medical implications, HIV/AIDS carries significant social and economic burdens. Stigma and discrimination towards people living with HIV persist globally, hindering prevention efforts and access to healthcare services. The disease disproportionately affects vulnerable populations, including men who have sex with men, sex workers, people who inject drugs, and marginalized communities, exacerbating social inequalities.

Research and Future Directions

Ongoing research focuses on developing an HIV vaccine, exploring novel treatment strategies such as long-acting antiretrovirals and gene therapy, and addressing persistent challenges in HIV cure research, including viral reservoirs and immune evasion mechanisms. Collaborative efforts between researchers, healthcare providers, policymakers, and affected communities remain essential to achieving the global goal of ending the HIV/AIDS epidemic by 2030, as outlined by the United Nations.

In conclusion, HIV & AIDS continue to pose significant challenges to global health, requiring a multifaceted approach encompassing prevention, treatment, research, and advocacy to mitigate their impact and ensure equitable access to care for all affected populations.

Epidemiology and Global Impact of HIV/AIDS

Human Immunodeficiency Virus (HIV) and Acquired Immunodeficiency Syndrome (AIDS) have profoundly impacted global health since their emergence in the early 1980s. This chapter explores the epidemiology of HIV/AIDS, its global distribution, key populations affected, socio-economic implications, and efforts towards prevention and control.

Historical Context and Emergence

The recognition of AIDS as a distinct clinical entity in the early 1980s marked the beginning of a global health crisis. Initially characterized by clusters of severe immune deficiency and opportunistic infections among previously healthy individuals, the identification of HIV as the causative agent in 1983 by researchers in France and the United States revolutionized understanding and response efforts.

Global Burden of HIV/AIDS

As of the latest estimates, approximately 37.7 million people globally were living with HIV in 2020. Despite significant progress in prevention and treatment efforts, the disease continues to pose substantial challenges, particularly in low- and middle-income countries. Sub-Saharan Africa remains the most heavily affected region, accounting for approximately two-thirds of all people living with HIV worldwide.

Epidemiological Trends

The epidemiology of HIV/AIDS exhibits significant regional and demographic variation. Key epidemiological indicators include HIV prevalence rates, incidence rates (new infections), mortality rates, and trends in key populations. Factors influencing these trends include socio-economic status, access to healthcare, cultural norms, and prevalence of risk behaviors such as unprotected sex and injecting drug use.

Regional Disparities

1. **Sub-Saharan Africa**: The epicenter of the HIV/AIDS pandemic, with high prevalence rates particularly among young women and girls. Structural factors such as poverty, gender inequality, and limited access to education and healthcare contribute to ongoing transmission.
2. **Asia**: Significant heterogeneity in HIV prevalence across countries, with concentrated epidemics among key populations including men who have sex with men (MSM), transgender individuals, people who inject drugs (PWID), and sex workers. Eastern Europe and Central Asia also experience growing epidemics linked to injecting drug use.
3. **Latin America and the Caribbean**: Varied epidemiological patterns ranging from generalized epidemics in some countries to concentrated epidemics among key populations in others. Socio-economic disparities and stigma remain significant barriers to prevention and treatment efforts.
4. **North America, Western and Central Europe**: Low to moderate prevalence overall, with stable or declining HIV incidence attributed to comprehensive prevention programs, widespread access to antiretroviral therapy (ART), and harm reduction strategies for key populations.

Key Populations Affected

Certain populations face disproportionately higher risks of HIV infection due to biological, behavioral, and structural factors:

- **Men who have sex with men (MSM)**: Globally, MSM are at significantly higher risk of HIV infection due to unprotected anal intercourse and stigma-driven barriers to healthcare access.
- **People who inject drugs (PWID)**: Sharing

contaminated needles and syringes contributes to high HIV prevalence among PWID, compounded by criminalization and marginalization.
- **Sex Workers**: Engagement in transactional sex without consistent condom use increases vulnerability to HIV infection, exacerbated by legal and social stigmatization.
- **Women and Girls**: Gender inequalities, including limited access to education and economic opportunities, heighten vulnerability to HIV infection among young women and girls, particularly in sub-Saharan Africa.

Socio-Economic and Health Impact

The socio-economic impact of HIV/AIDS extends beyond individual health outcomes to encompass broader economic and social dimensions:
- **Healthcare Systems**: Strain on healthcare systems due to increased demand for HIV-related services, including testing, treatment, and care for opportunistic infections.
- **Productivity and Workforce**: Loss of productivity and workforce participation due to morbidity and premature mortality among working-age adults, particularly in high-prevalence settings.
- **Family and Community Dynamics**: Disruption of family structures and caregiving responsibilities, with orphanhood and intergenerational impacts on children's well-being and development.

Prevention and Control Efforts

Effective HIV prevention and control strategies encompass a combination of biomedical, behavioral, and structural interventions:
- **Biomedical**: Promotion of HIV testing and counseling, access to antiretroviral therapy (ART) for treatment

and prevention (TasP), pre-exposure prophylaxis (PrEP) for high-risk individuals, and management of opportunistic infections.
- **Behavioral**: Promotion of safer sexual practices, harm reduction services for PWID, and educational initiatives to reduce stigma and discrimination.
- **Structural**: Addressing socio-economic determinants of health, including poverty, gender inequality, and legal barriers to healthcare access for key populations.

Global Response and Future Directions

The global response to HIV/AIDS has been characterized by unprecedented collaboration among governments, international organizations, civil society, and affected communities. Milestones include the United Nations' 90-90-90 targets, aimed at diagnosing 90% of all HIV-positive persons, providing ART to 90% of those diagnosed, and achieving viral suppression in 90% of those treated by 2020. Ongoing challenges include achieving equitable access to HIV services, addressing stigma and discrimination, and sustaining funding commitments for HIV/AIDS programs.

In conclusion, the epidemiology and global impact of HIV/AIDS underscore the urgent need for continued investment in prevention, treatment, and research efforts. Addressing socio-economic disparities, promoting human rights, and fostering inclusive health systems are essential to achieving the global goal of ending the HIV/AIDS epidemic by 2030, as articulated in the Sustainable Development Goals (SDGs).

Etiology and Pathogenesis of HIV

Human Immunodeficiency Virus (HIV) is a retrovirus that causes Acquired Immunodeficiency Syndrome (AIDS), a condition characterized by progressive immune system failure. Understanding the etiology and pathogenesis of HIV is crucial for developing effective treatments and prevention strategies.

HIV Structure and Function

HIV belongs to the family of Retroviridae and the genus Lentivirus. It is an enveloped virus with a lipid bilayer membrane derived from the host cell membrane. The viral envelope is studded with glycoprotein spikes composed of gp120 and gp41 proteins, which play essential roles in viral entry and fusion with host cells.

Viral Components

1. **Envelope (Env) Glycoprotein**: The surface of HIV is decorated with Env glycoproteins, gp120 and gp41. Gp120 binds to CD4 receptors on the surface of host cells, initiating the viral entry process.
2. **Capsid**: Inside the viral envelope lies the capsid, a protein shell that encloses the viral RNA genome and associated enzymes.
3. **RNA Genome**: HIV's genome is composed of two identical strands of positive-sense RNA, encoding essential viral proteins and regulatory elements.
4. **Reverse Transcriptase (RT)**: Upon entry into host cells, the virus uses its RT enzyme to convert its RNA genome into double-stranded DNA, a critical step in the viral replication cycle.
5. **Integrase**: Following reverse transcription, the viral DNA is integrated into the host cell genome by the viral integrase enzyme. Integration allows the virus to persist indefinitely within infected cells, forming latent viral reservoirs.
6. **Protease**: During viral maturation, the viral polyproteins produced by infected cells are cleaved into individual functional proteins by the viral protease enzyme, facilitating the assembly of new infectious viral particles.

HIV Life Cycle

The life cycle of HIV can be summarized into several key stages:

- **Attachment and Entry**: HIV initially binds to CD4 receptors on the surface of host cells (e.g., CD4 T-cells, macrophages) through gp120. This binding induces a conformational change in gp120, allowing it to interact with a co-receptor (either CCR5 or CXCR4), facilitating viral fusion and entry into the cell.
- **Reverse Transcription**: Once inside the host cell, the viral RNA genome is reverse transcribed into double-stranded DNA by the RT enzyme. The resulting viral DNA integrates into the host cell genome.
- **Integration**: Integrated viral DNA persists within the host cell nucleus, where it can remain latent or undergo transcription and translation to produce viral RNA and proteins.
- **Transcription and Translation**: Viral RNA is transcribed from the integrated DNA and serves as mRNA for the synthesis of viral proteins, including structural proteins (e.g., gag, pol, env) and regulatory proteins.
- **Assembly and Budding**: Viral proteins and RNA assemble at the host cell membrane, forming new viral particles that bud from the cell surface, acquiring an envelope containing host cell membrane proteins studded with viral glycoproteins.
- **Maturation**: Newly budded virions undergo maturation, during which viral protease cleaves the polyproteins into mature, functional proteins, rendering the virus infectious and ready to infect new target cells.

HIV Genetic Diversity and Drug Resistance

HIV exhibits high genetic diversity due to its error-prone reverse transcription process and rapid replication cycle. This genetic variability allows the virus to evade immune responses and develop resistance to antiretroviral drugs, posing challenges for treatment and vaccine development efforts.

Mechanism of HIV Transmission

HIV is primarily transmitted through contact with infected bodily fluids, most commonly:

- **Sexual Transmission**: Unprotected sexual intercourse, particularly anal and vaginal intercourse, is the predominant mode of HIV transmission worldwide. Transmission risk is higher in the presence of genital ulcerations, sexually transmitted infections (STIs), and high viral load in the infected partner.
- **Parenteral Transmission**: Transmission through contaminated needles and syringes among people who inject drugs (PWID) is a significant route of HIV transmission, particularly in settings where needle sharing is common.
- **Vertical Transmission**: HIV can be transmitted from an HIV-positive mother to her child during pregnancy, childbirth, or breastfeeding. Effective prevention of mother-to-child transmission (PMTCT) strategies, including antiretroviral therapy (ART) during pregnancy and breastfeeding, have significantly reduced transmission rates.
- **Blood Transfusion and Healthcare Settings**: Although rare in resource-rich settings due to stringent blood screening protocols, HIV transmission through contaminated blood products or medical procedures remains a concern in resource-limited settings with inadequate infection control measures.

Immune System Interaction

HIV infection profoundly impacts the immune system, targeting and impairing key components of both innate and adaptive immunity:

Impact on CD4 T-Cells

CD4 T-helper cells play a central role in coordinating immune responses and are primary targets for HIV infection. HIV-mediated depletion of CD4 cells leads to progressive immune dysfunction and susceptibility to opportunistic infections and cancers characteristic of AIDS.

- **Direct Cytopathic Effect**: HIV induces direct cytopathic effects on infected CD4 cells, causing cell death through viral replication, cell lysis, and apoptosis.
- **Immune Activation and Dysfunction**: Persistent immune activation, characterized by elevated levels of immune activation markers (e.g., CD38, HLA-DR) and inflammatory cytokines (e.g., TNF-alpha, IL-6), contributes to CD4 cell depletion and immune dysfunction.

Impact on Innate Immunity

HIV infection also affects innate immune cells, including macrophages and dendritic cells:

- **Macrophages**: HIV can infect and replicate within tissue-resident macrophages, contributing to viral persistence and chronic inflammation in tissues such as lymph nodes and the central nervous system.
- **Dendritic Cells**: HIV exploits dendritic cells as Trojan horses for viral dissemination to CD4 T-cells, enhancing viral spread and immune evasion strategies.

Immune Evasion Mechanisms

HIV employs several immune evasion strategies to evade host immune responses and establish persistent infection:

- **Antigenic Variation**: High mutation rates during viral replication allow HIV to evade neutralizing antibodies and cytotoxic T lymphocyte (CTL) responses by

generating diverse viral quasispecies.
- **Latency and Reservoir Formation**: HIV establishes latent reservoirs within long-lived memory CD4 T-cells, macrophages, and other tissue reservoirs (e.g., brain, gut-associated lymphoid tissue), evading immune surveillance and persisting despite effective ART.

Chronic Immune Activation and Inflammation

Chronic immune activation and inflammation are hallmarks of untreated HIV infection and contribute to disease progression and non-AIDS complications:
- **Microbial Translocation**: HIV-induced disruption of gut mucosal integrity leads to microbial translocation, allowing microbial products (e.g., lipopolysaccharide) to enter systemic circulation, fueling chronic inflammation and immune activation.
- **Co-Infections and Comorbidities**: Chronic immune activation predisposes individuals with HIV to increased risk of non-AIDS comorbidities, including cardiovascular disease, neurocognitive impairment, and certain cancers.

Immune Reconstitution and ART

Antiretroviral therapy (ART) suppresses viral replication, allowing immune reconstitution and partial restoration of immune function:
- **CD4 T-Cell Recovery**: ART-mediated suppression of viral replication enables gradual recovery of CD4 T-cell counts and reduction in immune activation markers, enhancing immune surveillance and reducing the risk of opportunistic infections.
- **Persistent Challenges**: Despite ART, residual immune dysfunction, including suboptimal CD4 T-cell recovery, persistent immune activation, and inflammation, contributes to increased morbidity and

mortality among people living with HIV.

Conclusion

In summary, HIV's etiology and pathogenesis involve intricate interactions between the virus and the host immune system, leading to progressive immune dysfunction and clinical manifestations of AIDS. A comprehensive understanding of HIV's structure, transmission dynamics, and immune evasion strategies is essential for developing effective therapies, preventive vaccines, and strategies to achieve long-term control and eradication of the virus. Continued research efforts and global collaboration are crucial in the ongoing fight against HIV/AIDS, aiming to improve outcomes for affected individuals and communities worldwide.

CHAPTER 2: HIV VIROLOGY AND BIOCHEMISTRY

HIV Types and Strains

Human Immunodeficiency Virus (HIV) is a highly diverse virus that exhibits considerable genetic variability, leading to distinct types and strains with varying geographic distributions and biological properties. Understanding the classification and diversity of HIV is essential for epidemiological surveillance, diagnostics, treatment selection, and vaccine development efforts.

Classification of HIV

HIV is classified into two main types, HIV-1 and HIV-2, each with distinct genetic and epidemiological characteristics:

HIV-1

HIV-1 is the predominant and most globally distributed type of HIV, responsible for the majority of HIV infections worldwide. It is further categorized into multiple groups, subtypes, and circulating recombinant forms (CRFs), reflecting its high genetic diversity and evolutionary dynamics.

HIV-1 Groups

1. **Group M (Main):** Group M viruses are responsible for the global HIV pandemic and can be further subdivided into subtypes (A-D, F-H, J, K) and numerous CRFs. Subtype B predominates in North America,

Europe, and Australia, whereas subtypes A, C, and D are prevalent in sub-Saharan Africa, India, and parts of Asia.

2. **Group O (Outlier)**: Group O viruses are primarily found in west-central Africa and represent a minority of HIV infections globally. They exhibit genetic differences from Group M viruses and pose challenges for diagnostic assays designed for Group M variants.
3. **Group N**: Group N viruses are rare and primarily confined to west-central Africa. They share ancestry with Group M viruses but exhibit distinct genetic differences.

HIV-1 Genetic Diversity

HIV-1's genetic diversity arises from its high mutation rate during replication, coupled with recombination events between different viral subtypes co-infecting the same host. Recombination contributes to the emergence of CRFs, which combine genetic segments from different subtypes and can exhibit unique biological properties or altered drug susceptibility.

HIV-2

HIV-2 is less prevalent and predominantly found in West Africa, particularly in countries such as Senegal, Guinea-Bissau, and Ivory Coast. It is genetically distinct from HIV-1 and generally exhibits slower disease progression. HIV-2 is classified into several subtypes (A-H), with subtype A and B being the most common.

Genetic and Biological Variability

The genetic variability of HIV has significant implications for disease progression, transmission dynamics, diagnosis, treatment outcomes, and vaccine development:

Disease Progression

- **HIV-1 Subtypes**: Some studies suggest that certain

HIV-1 subtypes, such as subtype D, may be associated with faster disease progression compared to others. Subtype B, prevalent in Western countries, historically exhibited more rapid progression to AIDS before the advent of effective antiretroviral therapy (ART).

- **HIV-2**: HIV-2 infections generally progress more slowly than HIV-1 infections, with a longer asymptomatic phase and delayed onset of AIDS-related complications. This difference in disease course is attributed to inherent differences in viral replication dynamics and immune responses.

Transmission Dynamics

- **Geographic Distribution**: The distribution of HIV-1 subtypes and CRFs varies geographically, influencing regional transmission dynamics and epidemic patterns. Subtype B predominates in North America and Western Europe, whereas subtypes A, C, and D are more prevalent in sub-Saharan Africa.
- **Transmission Fitness**: Viral fitness refers to the ability of a virus to replicate and spread within a host or population. Variations in viral fitness among different HIV subtypes and strains can impact transmission efficiency and epidemic dynamics.

Diagnostic and Treatment Considerations

- **Diagnostic Challenges**: The genetic diversity of HIV poses challenges for diagnostic assays designed to detect viral RNA or antibodies. Assays must be sensitive to detect diverse HIV variants and differentiate between HIV-1 and HIV-2 infections.
- **Treatment Response**: Antiretroviral drugs targeting specific viral proteins (e.g., protease, reverse transcriptase, integrase) may exhibit differential efficacy against various HIV subtypes and drug-resistant variants. Treatment selection often considers

viral genotype and resistance testing to optimize therapeutic outcomes.

Implications for Vaccine Development

The genetic diversity of HIV presents formidable challenges for developing an effective HIV vaccine capable of inducing broad and durable immune responses:

- **Vaccine Targets**: Vaccines typically target conserved regions of viral proteins critical for viral entry, replication, or immune evasion. The variability of HIV's envelope glycoproteins (gp120, gp41) necessitates the design of vaccines capable of eliciting cross-reactive neutralizing antibodies against diverse HIV strains.
- **Immune Responses**: HIV vaccines must induce robust cellular and humoral immune responses capable of neutralizing a broad spectrum of viral variants and preventing establishment of latent viral reservoirs.
- **Vaccine Trials**: Clinical trials of HIV vaccine candidates often involve diverse populations and evaluate vaccine efficacy against prevalent HIV subtypes and circulating strains. Vaccine development efforts continue to explore novel vaccine platforms, immunization strategies, and approaches to overcome HIV's genetic variability.

Conclusion

In conclusion, the classification and genetic diversity of HIV-1 and HIV-2 encompass a complex landscape of viral subtypes, strains, and recombinant forms with distinct epidemiological, biological, and clinical implications. Understanding HIV's genetic variability is essential for informing public health strategies, diagnostic approaches, treatment decisions, and ongoing efforts towards developing an effective HIV vaccine. Continued research into HIV's evolutionary dynamics and immune interactions is critical for advancing HIV prevention, treatment, and ultimately achieving global control of the HIV/AIDS pandemic.

Viral Life Cycle of HIV

Human Immunodeficiency Virus (HIV) is a retrovirus that infects and replicates within host cells, primarily CD4 T-cells and macrophages, leading to progressive immune dysfunction and ultimately Acquired Immunodeficiency Syndrome (AIDS). The viral life cycle of HIV is a complex and orchestrated series of events involving viral attachment, entry, reverse transcription, integration into the host genome, replication, assembly, budding, and maturation. Each stage of the HIV life cycle presents unique opportunities for therapeutic intervention and poses challenges for eradication efforts due to the establishment of latent viral reservoirs. This comprehensive review explores the molecular mechanisms and biological processes underlying the HIV life cycle.

Attachment and Entry

The initial steps of the HIV life cycle involve attachment of the virus to host cells, receptor binding, and fusion with the host cell membrane.

Viral Attachment:

1. **Attachment Factors**: HIV initially interacts with attachment factors on the surface of target cells, facilitating initial contact and concentration of virions near potential host cell receptors.
2. **CD4 Binding**: The viral envelope glycoprotein gp120 binds to the CD4 receptor on the surface of host cells, initiating the viral entry process. CD4 is primarily expressed on CD4 T-helper cells, macrophages, and dendritic cells.
3. **Co-Receptor Binding**: Following CD4 binding, conformational changes in gp120 enable interaction

with a co-receptor, typically either CCR5 or CXCR4. This interaction is crucial for the subsequent fusion of viral and cellular membranes.

Viral Fusion and Entry:

1. **Fusion Process**: The fusion process involves the insertion of the viral envelope into the host cell membrane, followed by merging of the lipid bilayers and release of the viral core into the host cell cytoplasm.
2. **Fusion Inhibitors**: Entry inhibitors, such as maraviroc, block the interaction between gp120 and CCR5, preventing viral fusion and entry into host cells. These inhibitors are used as part of antiretroviral therapy (ART) to prevent viral replication.

Reverse Transcription

Upon entry into the host cell, HIV undergoes reverse transcription, converting its single-stranded RNA genome into double-stranded DNA.

Reverse Transcription Process:

1. **Reverse Transcriptase (RT)**: The viral enzyme RT catalyzes the synthesis of a complementary DNA strand (cDNA) using the viral RNA genome as a template. RT possesses both RNA-dependent DNA polymerase activity (synthesis of DNA from RNA template) and DNA-dependent DNA polymerase activity (synthesis of second DNA strand).
2. **Generation of Proviral DNA**: Reverse transcription produces a double-stranded DNA molecule known as the proviral DNA, which consists of two identical DNA strands flanked by long terminal repeats (LTRs) derived from the viral RNA genome.
3. **RT Inhibitors**: Nucleoside/nucleotide RT inhibitors (NRTIs) and non-nucleoside RT inhibitors (NNRTIs) target the enzymatic activity of RT, preventing

the synthesis of proviral DNA. These drugs are essential components of ART regimens to inhibit viral replication.

Integration and Latency

Following reverse transcription, the proviral DNA integrates into the host cell genome, establishing a persistent reservoir of HIV-infected cells capable of long-term viral persistence.

Integration Process:

1. **Integration Machinery**: The integration of proviral DNA into the host genome is mediated by the viral enzyme integrase. Integrase catalyzes the cleavage of host cell DNA and the covalent attachment of proviral DNA ends to the host genome, forming integrated proviral DNA.
2. **Integration Site Preferences**: HIV integrates preferentially into actively transcribed regions of the host genome, such as near transcription start sites and within gene-rich regions. Integration site selection influences viral gene expression, replication competence, and persistence of infected cells.

Latency and Reservoir Formation:

1. **Latent Reservoirs**: Integrated proviral DNA can remain transcriptionally silent or latent within long-lived memory CD4 T-cells, macrophages, and other cell types. Latently infected cells evade immune surveillance and ART, contributing to viral persistence and rebound upon treatment interruption.
2. **Strategies to Target Latency**: Eradicating latent reservoirs remains a major challenge in HIV cure research. Strategies under investigation include latency-reversing agents (LRAs) to activate latent HIV expression, immune-mediated clearance of infected cells, and gene editing approaches to disrupt integrated proviral DNA.

Replication and Assembly

Once integrated into the host genome, HIV utilizes host cell machinery to transcribe viral RNA, translate viral proteins, and assemble new viral particles.

Viral Replication Cycle:

1. **Transcription and Translation**: The integrated proviral DNA serves as a template for transcription of viral RNA by host RNA polymerase II. Viral RNA transcripts encode viral structural proteins (Gag, Pol, Env), regulatory proteins (Tat, Rev), and accessory proteins (Vif, Vpr, Vpu, Nef).
2. **Protein Synthesis**: Viral RNA transcripts are translated into polyproteins, which are cleaved by viral protease into functional proteins essential for viral assembly and maturation.

Assembly of Viral Particles:

1. **Gag Polyprotein**: Gag polyproteins, translated from viral RNA, interact with viral RNA genomes to form the viral core. Gag proteins also recruit host cell membrane proteins and viral envelope glycoproteins (Env) to assembly sites at the host cell membrane.
2. **Budding Process**: Assembled viral cores bud through the host cell membrane, acquiring an envelope derived from the host cell membrane embedded with viral glycoproteins (gp120, gp41). The budding process is facilitated by interactions between Gag proteins and cellular ESCRT complexes.

Budding and Maturation

Following budding, immature viral particles undergo maturation, during which viral protease cleaves Gag and Gag-Pol polyproteins into individual structural proteins, rendering the virus infectious.

Maturation Process:

1. **Viral Protease Activation**: The viral protease enzyme becomes active within newly budded virions, cleaving Gag and Gag-Pol polyproteins at specific sites to generate mature viral proteins, including matrix (MA), capsid (CA), nucleocapsid (NC), and integrase (IN).
2. **Formation of Mature Virions**: Proteolytic cleavage of Gag polyprotein induces structural rearrangements within the viral core, promoting condensation and stabilization of the mature viral particle. Mature virions are released from the host cell and are now infectious, capable of initiating new rounds of infection in susceptible target cells.

Therapeutic Implications and Future Directions

Understanding the molecular mechanisms and biological processes underlying the HIV life cycle is critical for developing effective antiretroviral therapies, preventing viral transmission, and pursuing strategies for HIV cure and eradication:

- **Antiretroviral Therapy (ART)**: ART suppresses viral replication by targeting different stages of the HIV life cycle, including entry, reverse transcription, integration, and maturation. Combination ART (cART) regimens are highly effective in reducing viral load, preserving immune function, and improving clinical outcomes for people living with HIV.
- **HIV Cure Research**: Eradicating latent HIV reservoirs remains a major hurdle in achieving a functional cure for HIV/AIDS. Novel therapeutic approaches, including LRAs, immune-based therapies, and gene editing technologies (e.g., CRISPR/Cas9), are being investigated to achieve sustained virological remission or viral eradication.
- **Vaccine Development**: Insights into the HIV life cycle inform vaccine design strategies aimed at inducing protective immune responses against diverse HIV

strains. Ongoing efforts focus on eliciting broadly neutralizing antibodies (bnAbs) and cellular immune responses capable of controlling viral replication and preventing HIV infection.

Conclusion

In conclusion, the HIV life cycle is a dynamic and complex process involving sequential stages of viral attachment, entry, reverse transcription, integration, replication, assembly, budding, and maturation within host cells. Each stage of the HIV life cycle presents unique opportunities and challenges for therapeutic intervention, cure research, and vaccine development efforts. Continued research into the molecular mechanisms of HIV pathogenesis, viral-host interactions, and viral evolution is essential for advancing our understanding of HIV/AIDS and improving clinical outcomes for affected individuals worldwide.

Viral Mutability and Drug Resistance in HIV

Human Immunodeficiency Virus (HIV) is renowned for its high mutation rate and ability to develop resistance to antiretroviral therapies (ART), posing significant challenges in the management and treatment of HIV/AIDS. This section explores the mechanisms of viral mutability, factors influencing drug resistance development, clinical implications, and strategies to address these challenges.

Viral Mutability and Drug Resistance

Mechanisms of Viral Mutability

HIV's rapid evolution and genetic diversity are driven by several mechanisms inherent to its replication cycle:

Error-Prone Reverse Transcription

1. **Reverse Transcriptase (RT)**: During reverse transcription, HIV's RNA genome is converted into double-stranded DNA by RT. RT lacks proofreading

activity, resulting in a high error rate (approximately 1 error per 10,000 nucleotides incorporated). This error-prone process generates genetic diversity, giving rise to viral quasispecies within an infected individual.

2. **Quasispecies Formation**: HIV exists as a swarm of related but genetically distinct variants (quasispecies) within an infected individual. Quasispecies diversity allows the virus to adapt to selective pressures, evade immune responses, and develop resistance to antiretroviral drugs.

Recombination

1. **Recombination Events**: HIV's genome is prone to recombination during dual infection of a host cell by different viral strains. Recombination events between genetically distinct HIV variants can generate recombinant viruses with novel genetic characteristics, potentially impacting viral fitness and drug susceptibility.

Immune Selection Pressure

1. **Immune Escape Mutations**: Host immune responses exert selective pressure on HIV, favoring the emergence of mutations that reduce viral recognition and clearance by neutralizing antibodies or cytotoxic T lymphocytes (CTLs). Immune escape mutations contribute to ongoing viral replication and persistence despite immune surveillance.

Latency and Reservoir Dynamics

1. **Reservoir Diversity**: Latently infected cells, particularly long-lived memory CD4 T-cells and tissue macrophages, harbor integrated proviral DNA that can persist for years despite effective ART. The presence of diverse viral variants within latent reservoirs contributes to ongoing viral persistence and potential reactivation upon treatment interruption.

Factors Influencing Drug Resistance Development

HIV's ability to develop resistance to antiretroviral drugs is influenced by various factors, including viral replication dynamics, drug exposure, adherence to treatment regimens, and host immune status:

Viral Replication Dynamics

1. **High Replication Rate**: HIV replicates rapidly, producing billions of new viral particles daily. The sheer number of virions and the error-prone nature of RT increase the probability of acquiring mutations that confer resistance to antiretroviral drugs.
2. **Generation Time**: HIV has a short generation time (approximately 1-2 days), allowing rapid accumulation of mutations that may confer a selective advantage in the presence of antiretroviral drugs.

Drug Exposure and Adherence

1. **Suboptimal Drug Levels**: Inadequate drug exposure due to suboptimal adherence, drug interactions, or pharmacokinetic variability can result in subtherapeutic drug concentrations. Suboptimal drug levels promote viral replication and increase the likelihood of selecting for drug-resistant variants.
2. **Adherence Challenges**: Adherence to complex ART regimens is critical for maintaining sustained viral suppression and preventing the emergence of drug resistance. Factors influencing adherence include pill burden, regimen complexity, adverse effects, socioeconomic factors, and psychosocial support.

Drug Class and Resistance Pathways

1. **Resistance Mechanisms**: HIV develops resistance to antiretroviral drugs through several mechanisms, including mutations that alter drug binding sites (e.g., reverse transcriptase, protease, integrase), reduce drug

susceptibility, or enhance viral replication capacity in the presence of drugs.

2. **Cross-Resistance**: Some resistance mutations confer cross-resistance to multiple drugs within the same class (e.g., NNRTIs, NRTIs) or between different classes (e.g., NNRTIs and integrase strand transfer inhibitors [INSTIs]), limiting treatment options and complicating therapeutic management.

Host Immune Status

1. **Immune Deficiency**: Advanced HIV disease with low CD4 T-cell counts and impaired immune function correlates with higher viral replication rates and increased risk of developing drug resistance mutations.

2. **Immune Restoration**: Effective ART restores immune function and reduces HIV-associated immune activation, potentially enhancing immune surveillance and controlling viral replication. However, persistent immune activation and inflammation may contribute to ongoing viral replication and resistance development.

Clinical Implications of Drug Resistance

Drug-resistant HIV variants have significant clinical implications for HIV management, treatment outcomes, and public health:

Treatment Failure and Virological Rebound

1. **Virological Failure**: Inadequately treated HIV infections or suboptimal adherence may lead to virological failure, characterized by incomplete viral suppression and persistent viremia. Virological failure increases the risk of disease progression, opportunistic infections, and mortality.

2. **Virological Rebound**: Treatment interruptions or suboptimal adherence can result in virological

rebound, with rapid re-emergence of replication-competent HIV variants, including drug-resistant strains. Virological rebound necessitates regimen changes to restore viral suppression and prevent further resistance accumulation.

Limited Treatment Options

1. **Resistance Profiles**: The emergence of multidrug-resistant HIV strains limits treatment options and compromises the efficacy of standard ART regimens. Individuals with extensive drug resistance may require salvage therapies comprising newer antiretroviral agents with distinct resistance profiles and mechanisms of action.

2. **Individualized Treatment Strategies**: Resistance testing (genotypic or phenotypic) guides the selection of antiretroviral drugs based on individual resistance profiles, viral tropism, and treatment history. Individualized treatment strategies optimize therapeutic outcomes and minimize the risk of further resistance development.

Public Health Challenges

1. **Transmission of Drug-Resistant HIV**: Drug-resistant HIV strains can be transmitted to newly infected individuals, contributing to primary drug resistance and complicating initial treatment choices. Enhanced surveillance, early diagnosis, and prompt initiation of effective ART are essential for controlling drug-resistant HIV transmission.

2. **Healthcare Costs and Resource Allocation**: Managing drug-resistant HIV strains requires costly antiretroviral regimens, resistance testing, and comprehensive clinical monitoring. Healthcare systems must allocate resources to support sustainable HIV care, treatment access, and adherence

support services.

Strategies to Address Drug Resistance

Addressing HIV drug resistance requires a multifaceted approach encompassing prevention strategies, enhanced surveillance, adherence support, novel treatment development, and global collaboration:

Prevention Strategies

1. **Early Diagnosis and Treatment**: Early diagnosis of HIV infection and prompt initiation of ART reduce viral replication, preserve immune function, and minimize the risk of developing drug resistance.
2. **Pre-Exposure Prophylaxis (PrEP)**: PrEP with antiretroviral drugs, such as tenofovir/emtricitabine, prevents HIV acquisition among at-risk individuals and reduces the transmission of drug-resistant HIV strains.

Enhanced Surveillance and Monitoring

1. **Resistance Testing**: Routine genotypic or phenotypic resistance testing informs treatment decisions and identifies emerging drug resistance mutations. Access to resistance testing facilitates personalized treatment strategies and surveillance of resistance trends.
2. **Surveillance Programs**: National and global surveillance programs monitor the prevalence of drug-resistant HIV strains, assess treatment outcomes, and inform public health policies to mitigate transmission and optimize treatment regimens.

Adherence Support and Patient Education

1. **Adherence Counseling**: Comprehensive adherence support services, including counseling, pillbox organizers, reminder tools, and mobile health technologies, promote sustained adherence to ART regimens and minimize the risk of treatment failure.

2. **Patient Education**: Educating individuals living with HIV about the importance of adherence, drug resistance, and treatment options enhances treatment literacy, empowers patient decision-making, and improves long-term clinical outcomes.

Novel Antiretroviral Therapies and Combinations

1. **Next-Generation Antiretrovirals**: Continued research and development of novel antiretroviral drugs with distinct resistance profiles, improved tolerability, and enhanced potency against drug-resistant HIV variants expand treatment options and support salvage therapy strategies.
2. **Combination Therapies**: Tailoring ART regimens with multiple drugs targeting different stages of the HIV life cycle (e.g., protease inhibitors, integrase inhibitors, entry inhibitors) reduces the risk of resistance development and optimizes viral suppression in treatment-experienced individuals.

Global Collaboration and Research

1. **Research Initiatives**: Collaborative research efforts focus on understanding viral mutability, resistance mechanisms, and host-pathogen interactions to advance HIV cure strategies, develop long-acting antiretroviral formulations, and ultimately achieve sustained viral remission or eradication.
2. **International Guidelines and Policies**: International guidelines (e.g., WHO HIV treatment guidelines) provide evidence-based recommendations for antiretroviral therapy initiation, drug resistance testing, and management of drug-resistant HIV infections, promoting standardized care and treatment equity globally.

Conclusion

In conclusion, HIV's mutability and ability to develop resistance to antiretroviral drugs present ongoing challenges in the global fight against HIV/AIDS. Understanding the molecular mechanisms of viral mutability, factors influencing drug resistance development, and clinical implications is essential for optimizing HIV treatment outcomes, preventing transmission of drug-resistant strains, and advancing efforts towards HIV cure and eradication. Multifaceted strategies, including early diagnosis, adherence support, novel antiretroviral therapies, and global collaboration, are crucial for addressing HIV drug resistance and achieving long-term control of the HIV/AIDS pandemic. Continued research, innovation, and public health efforts are essential to mitigate the impact of drug-resistant HIV and improve the quality of life for individuals living with HIV worldwide.

Immunopathogenesis of HIV

The immunopathogenesis of Human Immunodeficiency Virus (HIV) infection involves intricate interactions between the virus and the host immune system, leading to progressive immune dysfunction and the development of Acquired Immunodeficiency Syndrome (AIDS). This section explores the underlying mechanisms of HIV-induced immunopathogenesis, including viral dynamics, immune responses, inflammation, and the implications for HIV management and therapeutic strategies.

Introduction to Immunopathogenesis

HIV infection is characterized by a progressive depletion of CD4 T-helper cells, impaired immune function, and chronic immune activation, ultimately resulting in immunodeficiency and increased susceptibility to opportunistic infections and malignancies. The pathogenesis of HIV involves a complex interplay between viral replication, immune responses, and inflammatory processes that contribute to both viral persistence and immune dysfunction.

Viral Dynamics in HIV Infection

The dynamics of HIV replication and viral reservoirs play a critical role in shaping the immunopathogenesis of HIV:

Viral Replication Cycles

1. **Replication in Target Cells**: HIV primarily infects CD4 T-cells, macrophages, and dendritic cells through receptor-mediated entry and fusion. Following entry, viral RNA is reverse transcribed into proviral DNA, which integrates into the host genome and undergoes transcription and translation to produce new viral particles.
2. **Viral Reservoirs**: Latently infected CD4 T-cells, particularly memory T-cells, harbor integrated proviral DNA that can persist for years despite effective antiretroviral therapy (ART). Viral reservoirs contribute to ongoing viral replication, rebound viremia upon treatment interruption, and challenges in achieving viral eradication or functional cure.

Immune Responses to HIV

1. **Cell-Mediated Immunity**: HIV-specific cytotoxic T lymphocytes (CTLs) recognize and eliminate HIV-infected cells through direct cytotoxicity and cytokine-mediated mechanisms. CTL responses contribute to the control of viral replication and containment of HIV reservoirs.
2. **Humoral Immunity**: Antibodies targeting HIV envelope glycoproteins (gp120, gp41) can neutralize viral particles and mediate antibody-dependent cellular cytotoxicity (ADCC). However, HIV's high mutation rate and structural variability pose challenges for eliciting broadly neutralizing antibodies effective against diverse viral strains.

Chronic Immune Activation

1. **Persistent Inflammation**: HIV infection induces chronic immune activation characterized by elevated levels of pro-inflammatory cytokines (e.g., IL-6, TNF-alpha), immune activation markers (e.g., CD38, HLA-DR), and coagulation markers (e.g., D-dimer). Chronic inflammation contributes to immune dysfunction, accelerated T-cell turnover, and increased cardiovascular and non-AIDS-related morbidity.
2. **Microbial Translocation**: HIV-related disruption of gut-associated lymphoid tissue (GALT) integrity leads to microbial translocation, with bacterial products (e.g., lipopolysaccharide, LPS) entering systemic circulation and triggering immune activation. Microbial translocation contributes to systemic inflammation, immune dysfunction, and disease progression in HIV-infected individuals.

Pathological Mechanisms of HIV Immunopathogenesis

The pathological mechanisms underlying HIV-induced immunopathogenesis involve direct viral effects, immune-mediated responses, and interactions between HIV and host immune cells:

CD4 T-Cell Depletion

1. **Direct Viral Cytopathicity**: HIV replicates within CD4 T-cells, leading to direct cytopathic effects, cell death (lytic infection), and progressive depletion of CD4 T-cell subsets essential for orchestrating immune responses.
2. **Syncytium Formation**: HIV envelope glycoproteins (gp120, gp41) facilitate cell-cell fusion, forming multinucleated giant cells (syncytia) that contribute to CD4 T-cell depletion and viral dissemination within lymphoid tissues.

Immune Dysregulation

1. **Loss of Regulatory T-Cells**: HIV disrupts regulatory

T-cell (Treg) function and homeostasis, impairing immune tolerance mechanisms and exacerbating immune activation and inflammation.
2. **Th17/Treg Imbalance**: HIV-mediated depletion of Th17 cells, which maintain mucosal barrier integrity and modulate immune responses, disrupts the balance between Th17 and Treg populations, contributing to gut mucosal damage and microbial translocation.

Dysfunctional Immune Responses
1. **Exhaustion of T-Cell Responses**: Prolonged exposure to high antigen loads and chronic immune activation lead to T-cell exhaustion characterized by reduced proliferation, cytokine production, and cytotoxic function, impairing HIV-specific immune responses.
2. **Impaired B-Cell Function**: HIV-associated B-cell dysfunction, including reduced antibody production, impaired class-switching, and altered B-cell repertoire, compromises humoral immune responses and limits the efficacy of vaccine-induced immunity.

Clinical Manifestations and Complications

HIV-induced immunopathogenesis manifests clinically through progressive immune dysfunction, opportunistic infections, and non-AIDS-related complications:

Opportunistic Infections
1. **Bacterial Infections**: HIV-associated immunodeficiency increases susceptibility to bacterial infections, including Mycobacterium tuberculosis, Streptococcus pneumoniae, and Salmonella species, contributing to high morbidity and mortality among untreated individuals.
2. **Fungal Infections**: Opportunistic fungal infections, such as Candida species and Pneumocystis jirovecii pneumonia (PCP), are common in advanced HIV disease with CD4 T-cell depletion and impaired cell-

mediated immunity.

Viral Infections

1. **Viral Opportunistic Infections**: HIV-related immune suppression predisposes individuals to viral opportunistic infections, including cytomegalovirus (CMV) retinitis, herpes simplex virus (HSV) infections, and progressive multifocal leukoencephalopathy (PML).
2. **Oncogenic Viruses**: Persistent infection with oncogenic viruses, such as human papillomavirus (HPV), Epstein-Barr virus (EBV), and hepatitis B virus (HBV), increases the risk of virus-associated cancers (e.g., cervical cancer, lymphoma) in HIV-infected individuals.

Non-AIDS-Related Complications

1. **Cardiovascular Disease**: Chronic inflammation, immune activation, and metabolic disturbances in HIV-infected individuals contribute to an increased risk of cardiovascular disease (CVD), myocardial infarction, and stroke.
2. **Neurocognitive Impairment**: HIV-associated neurocognitive disorders (HAND) encompass a spectrum of neurological deficits, ranging from mild cognitive impairment to severe HIV-associated dementia, influenced by viral neurotropism, chronic inflammation, and immune dysregulation.

Therapeutic Strategies and Future Directions

Optimizing therapeutic strategies for HIV management and addressing immunopathogenesis involve comprehensive approaches to suppress viral replication, restore immune function, and mitigate inflammatory responses:

Antiretroviral Therapy (ART)

1. **Suppressing Viral Replication**: Early initiation of

ART suppresses viral replication, preserves CD4 T-cell counts, and reduces HIV-associated immune activation and inflammation. Combination ART (cART) regimens comprising multiple antiretroviral drug classes effectively achieve sustained viral suppression and prevent disease progression.
2. **Immune Restoration**: Effective ART restores immune function, reduces chronic inflammation, and improves clinical outcomes for HIV-infected individuals. Immune-based therapies, including interleukin-7 (IL-7) and therapeutic vaccination strategies, aim to enhance immune reconstitution and control viral reservoirs.

Targeting Chronic Inflammation
1. **Anti-Inflammatory Therapies**: Adjunctive therapies targeting chronic inflammation in HIV, such as statins, anti-TNF agents, and anti-inflammatory cytokine blockers, may mitigate immune activation, reduce cardiovascular risk, and improve long-term health outcomes.
2. **Microbiome Interventions**: Interventions targeting gut microbiota composition and function, including probiotics, prebiotics, and microbial-based therapies, aim to restore gut mucosal integrity, reduce microbial translocation, and modulate systemic inflammation in HIV-infected individuals.

Cure Strategies and HIV Remission
1. **Viral Reservoir Eradication**: Cure research focuses on eradicating latent HIV reservoirs through latency-reversing agents (LRAs), immune-mediated clearance strategies, and gene editing technologies (e.g., CRISPR/Cas9) to achieve sustained virological remission or functional cure.
2. **Long-Acting Therapies**: Development of long-acting

antiretroviral formulations (e.g., injectable ART, implantable devices) aims to improve treatment adherence, reduce treatment fatigue, and optimize viral suppression and immune restoration in HIV-infected individuals.

Global Health Strategies

1. **Global Access to Treatment**: Universal access to affordable ART, diagnostic testing, and comprehensive HIV care services is essential for achieving global HIV treatment goals, reducing health disparities, and controlling the HIV/AIDS pandemic.
2. **Research and Innovation**: Continued investment in HIV research, innovation, and international collaboration is critical for advancing therapeutic strategies, developing novel antiretroviral drugs, understanding viral immunopathogenesis, and ultimately achieving sustained control of HIV infection worldwide.

Conclusion

In conclusion, HIV-induced immunopathogenesis involves complex interactions between viral replication, immune responses, chronic inflammation, and host immune dysfunction, culminating in progressive CD4 T-cell depletion, immune suppression, and increased susceptibility to opportunistic infections and non-AIDS-related complications. Understanding the mechanisms of HIV immunopathogenesis informs therapeutic strategies aimed at suppressing viral replication, restoring immune function, mitigating inflammation, and advancing efforts towards achieving HIV cure or sustained viral remission. Multidisciplinary approaches, including early diagnosis, optimized antiretroviral therapies, immune-based interventions, and global health strategies, are essential for addressing HIV immunopathogenesis, improving clinical outcomes, and mitigating the global impact of HIV/AIDS.

Continued research, innovation, and commitment to equity in healthcare access are critical for achieving long-term control and ultimately ending the HIV/AIDS pandemic.

CHAPTER 3: ANATOMY AND PHYSIOLOGY

Immune System Overview

The immune system is a complex network of organs, tissues, cells, and molecules that work together to defend the body against pathogens, such as bacteria, viruses, fungi, and parasites, and to maintain homeostasis. In the context of Human Immunodeficiency Virus (HIV) infection, understanding the structure, function, and interactions of the immune system is crucial for comprehending how HIV evades immune surveillance, induces immune dysfunction, and leads to progressive immunodeficiency and AIDS. This section provides an in-depth overview of the immune system, focusing on its components, functions, and implications for HIV pathogenesis and therapeutic strategies.

Introduction to the Immune System

The immune system comprises two main branches: the innate immune system and the adaptive (or acquired) immune system. Each branch plays distinct roles in recognizing and responding to pathogens, maintaining immune memory, and coordinating immune responses.

Innate Immune System

The innate immune system provides immediate, nonspecific defense mechanisms against pathogens:

1. **Physical Barriers**: Physical barriers, such as the skin and mucosal surfaces (e.g., respiratory, gastrointestinal, genitourinary tracts), prevent pathogen entry into the body and provide the first line of defense against infection.
2. **Cellular Components**: Innate immune cells include phagocytes (neutrophils, macrophages), natural killer (NK) cells, dendritic cells, and innate lymphoid cells. These cells detect and engulf pathogens through pattern recognition receptors (PRRs) recognizing conserved microbial structures (e.g., lipopolysaccharides, peptidoglycans).
3. **Inflammatory Responses**: Innate immune cells release cytokines, chemokines, and inflammatory mediators to recruit immune cells to the site of infection, enhance phagocytosis, and activate adaptive immune responses.

Adaptive Immune System

The adaptive immune system provides specific, long-lasting immunity against pathogens:

1. **Cellular Immunity**: T lymphocytes (T-cells) play central roles in cellular immunity. CD4 T-helper cells coordinate immune responses by secreting cytokines that activate other immune cells (e.g., B cells, macrophages, cytotoxic T cells). CD8 cytotoxic T cells recognize and kill infected cells through direct cytotoxicity.
2. **Humoral Immunity**: B lymphocytes (B cells) differentiate into plasma cells that produce antibodies (immunoglobulins) specific to antigens present on pathogens. Antibodies neutralize pathogens, promote phagocytosis through opsonization, and mediate antibody-dependent cellular cytotoxicity (ADCC).
3. **Immune Memory**: Both T and B cells develop

immunological memory following initial antigen exposure. Memory cells facilitate rapid and enhanced immune responses upon re-exposure to the same pathogen, contributing to long-term protective immunity.

Components of the Immune System

Cellular Components

1. **Leukocytes**: White blood cells (leukocytes) include granulocytes (neutrophils, eosinophils, basophils), monocytes (which differentiate into macrophages and dendritic cells), and lymphocytes (T cells, B cells, NK cells).
2. **Phagocytes**: Phagocytic cells, such as neutrophils and macrophages, engulf and digest pathogens and cellular debris through phagocytosis, promoting pathogen clearance and immune surveillance.
3. **Lymphocytes**: Lymphocytes circulate through the blood and lymphatic system, surveilling for antigens. T cells recognize antigens presented by major histocompatibility complex (MHC) molecules on infected cells, while B cells produce antibodies specific to antigens encountered.

Soluble Mediators

1. **Cytokines and Chemokines**: Cytokines are signaling proteins secreted by immune cells to regulate immune responses, inflammation, and hematopoiesis. Chemokines attract immune cells to sites of infection or inflammation.
2. **Complement System**: The complement system consists of circulating proteins that enhance opsonization, promote inflammation, and directly lyse pathogens through membrane attack complexes (MAC).
3. **Antibodies**: Immunoglobulins (IgG, IgA, IgM, IgE,

IgD) are antibodies produced by B cells that recognize and bind to specific antigens on pathogens, neutralizing them and marking them for destruction by phagocytes.

Functions of the Immune System

Recognition and Response to Pathogens

1. **Pattern Recognition Receptors (PRRs)**: PRRs, such as Toll-like receptors (TLRs) and NOD-like receptors (NLRs), detect conserved microbial patterns (e.g., lipopolysaccharides, viral RNA) and initiate innate immune responses.
2. **Antigen Presentation**: Antigen-presenting cells (APCs), including dendritic cells, macrophages, and B cells, capture, process, and present antigens to T cells via MHC molecules, initiating adaptive immune responses.
3. **Immune Activation**: Activated T cells secrete cytokines (e.g., IL-2, IFN-gamma) that regulate immune cell activation, proliferation, differentiation, and effector functions, coordinating immune responses against pathogens.

Immune Regulation and Tolerance

1. **Immune Tolerance**: Regulatory T cells (Tregs) maintain immune tolerance and prevent autoimmune reactions by suppressing excessive immune responses and maintaining self-tolerance to host tissues.
2. **Homeostasis**: The immune system maintains homeostasis through balanced immune activation and regulation, ensuring effective pathogen clearance while minimizing tissue damage and autoimmune responses.

Implications for HIV Pathogenesis

HIV Interaction with the Immune System

1. **CD4 T-Cell Targeting**: HIV targets CD4 T-cells, macrophages, and dendritic cells through CD4 receptor and co-receptors (e.g., CCR5, CXCR4), leading to direct viral infection, replication, and CD4 T-cell depletion.
2. **Immune Evasion Strategies**: HIV evades immune detection and elimination through mechanisms, including rapid mutation (escape from antibody recognition), latency in reservoirs (escape from CTL surveillance), and modulation of host immune responses.
3. **Chronic Immune Activation**: Persistent HIV replication and immune activation contribute to chronic inflammation, immune dysfunction, and exhaustion of HIV-specific immune responses, accelerating disease progression and immune system deterioration.

Therapeutic Strategies Targeting the Immune System

Antiretroviral Therapy (ART)

1. **Viral Suppression**: ART suppresses HIV replication, preserves CD4 T-cell counts, and restores immune function by reducing viral load, preventing opportunistic infections, and improving overall health outcomes.
2. **Immune Restoration**: Effective ART restores CD4 T-cell counts, reduces chronic immune activation and inflammation, and enhances immune reconstitution in HIV-infected individuals.

Immune-Based Therapies

1. **Interleukin Therapies**: Interleukin-2 (IL-2) therapy enhances immune responses and CD4 T-cell recovery in combination with ART, while IL-7 and IL-15 therapies promote T-cell survival and proliferation.

2. **Checkpoint Inhibitors**: Checkpoint inhibitors (e.g., anti-PD-1, anti-CTLA-4 antibodies) restore exhausted T-cell function, enhance immune responses against HIV-infected cells, and are under investigation for HIV cure strategies.

Vaccination Strategies

1. **Therapeutic Vaccines**: Therapeutic vaccines aim to stimulate HIV-specific immune responses, reduce viral reservoirs, and control viral replication in combination with ART, advancing efforts towards functional cure or remission.
2. **Preventive Vaccines**: Vaccine development targets HIV envelope glycoproteins (gp120, gp41) to induce broadly neutralizing antibodies and cellular immunity, potentially preventing HIV acquisition and transmission.

Conclusion

The immune system is a dynamic and intricate defense network essential for protecting the body against infections and maintaining health. In the context of HIV infection, HIV targets and disrupts immune responses, leading to progressive immune dysfunction, CD4 T-cell depletion, and susceptibility to opportunistic infections. Understanding the complexities of immune system interactions with HIV informs therapeutic strategies aimed at suppressing viral replication, restoring immune function, and advancing efforts towards HIV cure and long-term control. Continued research, innovation in immunotherapy, and global collaboration are crucial for achieving sustainable HIV management and improving outcomes for individuals living with HIV/AIDS worldwide.

CD4 T-Cell Biology and Function

CD4 T-cells, a subset of T lymphocytes expressing the CD4

receptor molecule, play pivotal roles in orchestrating adaptive immune responses, maintaining immune homeostasis, and coordinating defense against pathogens. In the context of Human Immunodeficiency Virus (HIV) infection, understanding CD4 T-cell biology and function is crucial as HIV specifically targets and depletes these cells, leading to profound immunodeficiency and progression to Acquired Immunodeficiency Syndrome (AIDS). This section provides a comprehensive exploration of CD4 T-cell biology, including their development, differentiation, activation, functions in immune responses, interactions with HIV, and implications for therapeutic interventions.

Introduction to CD4 T-Cells

CD4 T-cells are central players in the adaptive immune system, involved in recognizing peptide antigens presented by major histocompatibility complex class II (MHC-II) molecules on antigen-presenting cells (APCs). Upon activation, CD4 T-cells differentiate into various effector subsets that orchestrate immune responses tailored to combat specific pathogens and regulate immune functions.

Development and Differentiation of CD4 T-Cells

CD4 T-cell development begins in the thymus, where hematopoietic progenitor cells migrate and undergo differentiation under the influence of thymic stromal cells and cytokines. Key stages of CD4 T-cell development include:

1. **Thymic Selection**: Double-positive thymocytes expressing both CD4 and CD8 undergo positive and negative selection processes to generate mature single-positive CD4 or CD8 T-cells with diverse T-cell receptor (TCR) specificities.

2. **Peripheral Differentiation**: Naïve CD4 T-cells (CD4+CD45RA+CCR7+) circulate in peripheral blood and secondary lymphoid organs, where they encounter antigens presented by APCs. Antigen

recognition and co-stimulatory signals induce CD4 T-cell activation and differentiation into distinct effector subsets.

Effector Subsets of CD4 T-Cells

Activated CD4 T-cells differentiate into specialized effector subsets characterized by unique cytokine profiles and functions:

1. **Th1 Cells**: Th1 cells (producing IFN-gamma, TNF-alpha) mediate cellular immunity against intracellular pathogens (e.g., viruses, intracellular bacteria) by activating macrophages and cytotoxic T-cells.
2. **Th2 Cells**: Th2 cells (producing IL-4, IL-5, IL-13) promote humoral immunity, eosinophil activation, and antibody production, critical for defense against extracellular parasites and allergic responses.
3. **Th17 Cells**: Th17 cells (producing IL-17, IL-22) defend mucosal barriers against fungal and extracellular bacterial infections, regulate tissue inflammation, and maintain epithelial integrity.
4. **Treg Cells**: Regulatory T cells (Tregs, producing IL-10, TGF-beta) suppress excessive immune responses, maintain immune tolerance, and prevent autoimmune reactions by inhibiting effector T-cell function.
5. **Tfh Cells**: T follicular helper cells (Tfh, producing IL-21) provide B-cell help within germinal centers, promoting antibody class-switching, affinity maturation, and long-term humoral immunity.

Functions of CD4 T-Cells in Immune Responses

CD4 T-cells orchestrate immune responses through diverse mechanisms, integrating signals from APCs, co-stimulatory molecules, and cytokine microenvironments:

Antigen Recognition and Activation

1. **T-Cell Receptor Signaling**: Interaction between TCRs and peptide-MHC complexes on APCs triggers

intracellular signaling pathways, leading to CD4 T-cell activation, proliferation, and differentiation into effector or memory T-cells.

2. **Co-Stimulatory Signals**: Co-stimulatory molecules (e.g., CD28, CD40 ligand) provide additional signals required for full T-cell activation, cytokine production, and differentiation into effector subsets tailored to combat specific pathogens.

Cytokine Production and Immune Regulation

1. **Cytokine Secretion**: Activated CD4 T-cells secrete cytokines (e.g., IFN-gamma, IL-2, IL-4) that regulate immune responses, activate other immune cells (e.g., macrophages, B cells), and modulate inflammation and tissue repair processes.

2. **Immune Modulation**: Th1, Th2, Th17, Treg, and Tfh subsets exert context-dependent immune modulatory effects, shaping immune responses against pathogens, maintaining immune tolerance, and regulating tissue homeostasis.

Memory T-Cell Responses

1. **Formation of Memory T-Cells**: Following antigen encounter and clonal expansion, a subset of activated CD4 T-cells differentiate into long-lived memory T-cells (central memory T-cells, Tcm; effector memory T-cells, Tem) capable of rapid and robust recall responses upon re-exposure to specific antigens.

2. **Protective Immunity**: Memory CD4 T-cells contribute to long-term protective immunity by facilitating rapid cytokine production, activation of effector cells, and enhancement of secondary immune responses against previously encountered pathogens.

CD4 T-Cells in HIV Pathogenesis

HIV infection critically targets and disrupts CD4 T-cell functions, leading to profound immune dysfunction and immunodeficiency:

Mechanisms of CD4 T-Cell Depletion

1. **Direct HIV Infection**: HIV primarily infects CD4 T-cells through interaction with CD4 receptors and co-receptors (e.g., CCR5, CXCR4), leading to viral replication, cytopathic effects, and CD4 T-cell death (lytic infection).
2. **Syncytium Formation**: HIV envelope glycoproteins (gp120, gp41) facilitate cell-cell fusion and syncytium formation, contributing to massive CD4 T-cell depletion, immune activation, and viral dissemination within lymphoid tissues.

Immune Dysfunction and Exhaustion

1. **Progressive CD4 T-Cell Decline**: Chronic HIV replication and viral persistence in lymphoid tissues accelerate CD4 T-cell depletion, impairing immune surveillance, and reducing capacity for effective immune responses against opportunistic infections.
2. **Immune Exhaustion**: Prolonged exposure to high viral antigen loads induces functional exhaustion of HIV-specific CD4 T-cells, characterized by reduced cytokine production, proliferation, and cytotoxic capacity, contributing to immune dysfunction and disease progression.

Therapeutic Strategies Targeting CD4 T-Cells

Understanding CD4 T-cell biology informs therapeutic approaches aimed at preserving immune function, enhancing immune responses, and mitigating HIV-associated immune dysfunction:

Antiretroviral Therapy (ART)

1. **Preserving CD4 T-Cell Counts**: Early initiation of ART suppresses HIV replication, preserves CD4 T-cell counts, and restores immune function, reducing the

risk of opportunistic infections and improving long-term clinical outcomes.

2. **Immune Reconstitution**: Effective ART promotes CD4 T-cell recovery, reduces immune activation and inflammation, and enhances the restoration of HIV-specific immune responses, supporting immune reconstitution in HIV-infected individuals.

Immune-Based Interventions

1. **Cytokine Therapies**: Interleukin therapies (e.g., IL-2, IL-7) enhance CD4 T-cell survival, proliferation, and immune reconstitution in combination with ART, potentially optimizing therapeutic outcomes and immune responses.

2. **Checkpoint Inhibitors**: Immune checkpoint inhibitors (e.g., anti-PD-1, anti-CTLA-4 antibodies) reverse CD4 T-cell exhaustion, restore immune function, and augment immune responses against persistent HIV infection, under investigation for HIV cure strategies.

Vaccination Strategies

1. **Therapeutic Vaccines**: Therapeutic vaccines targeting HIV antigens aim to boost HIV-specific CD4 T-cell responses, reduce viral reservoirs, and enhance immune control of viral replication in combination with ART, advancing efforts towards functional HIV cure or remission.

2. **Preventive Vaccines**: Vaccine development strategies targeting HIV envelope glycoproteins (gp120, gp41) aim to induce broadly neutralizing antibodies and CD4 T-cell responses, potentially preventing HIV acquisition and transmission in at-risk populations.

Conclusion

CD4 T-cells are essential regulators of adaptive immune responses, contributing to immune surveillance, pathogen clearance, and immune memory formation. In HIV infection,

CD4 T-cells are primary targets of viral infection and depletion, leading to progressive immunodeficiency and increased susceptibility to opportunistic infections. Understanding CD4 T-cell biology and function provides insights into HIV pathogenesis, immune dysfunction, and therapeutic strategies aimed at preserving immune function, restoring immune responses, and advancing efforts towards HIV cure or sustained control. Continued research, innovation in immunotherapy, and global collaboration are critical for improving HIV treatment outcomes and addressing the global impact of HIV/AIDS.

Lymphatic System Involvement in HIV/AIDS

The lymphatic system plays a crucial role in immune surveillance, fluid balance, and the transport of immune cells and antigens throughout the body. In the context of Human Immunodeficiency Virus (HIV) infection, the lymphatic system becomes intricately involved in HIV pathogenesis, dissemination, immune response modulation, and disease progression. This section provides a comprehensive exploration of the lymphatic system's anatomy, functions, interactions with HIV, and implications for HIV/AIDS pathophysiology and clinical management.

Anatomy and Functions of the Lymphatic System

The lymphatic system consists of a network of lymphatic vessels, lymph nodes, lymphoid organs (e.g., spleen, thymus, tonsils), and lymphatic tissues (e.g., mucosa-associated lymphoid tissue, MALT) distributed throughout the body. Key components include:

Lymphatic Vessels

Lymphatic vessels are thin-walled tubes that parallel blood vessels, carrying lymph—a clear, protein-rich fluid derived from interstitial fluid and cellular debris. Lymphatic capillaries absorb excess tissue fluid, proteins, lipids, and immune cells from tissues, transporting them to lymph nodes for filtration and immune surveillance.

Lymph Nodes

Lymph nodes are encapsulated organs located along lymphatic vessels, acting as filtering stations where antigens and immune cells interact. Lymph nodes contain lymphoid tissue, including B cells, T cells, macrophages, and dendritic cells, facilitating immune responses against pathogens and antigens present in lymph.

Lymphoid Organs and Tissues

Beyond lymph nodes, lymphoid organs (e.g., spleen, thymus) and tissues (e.g., MALT in gastrointestinal tract, tonsils in upper respiratory tract) contribute to immune surveillance, antigen presentation, and immune cell maturation, supporting systemic immune responses and maintaining immune homeostasis.

HIV Interaction with the Lymphatic System

Lymphoid Tissue Reservoirs

HIV targets lymphoid tissues rich in CD4 T-cells, macrophages, and dendritic cells, establishing viral reservoirs and promoting viral replication, persistence, and dissemination:

1. **Primary Infection Sites**: HIV initially infects CD4 T-cells and macrophages within mucosal tissues (e.g., gut-associated lymphoid tissue, GALT) and secondary lymphoid organs (e.g., lymph nodes), facilitating systemic viral spread and seeding of lymphoid reservoirs.
2. **Viral Reservoirs**: Lymphoid tissues serve as sanctuary sites for HIV, shielding infected cells from immune surveillance and antiretroviral therapy (ART), contributing to viral persistence, latent infection, and potential viral rebound upon treatment interruption.

Immune Activation and Dysfunction

1. **Chronic Immune Activation**: HIV-induced immune activation within lymphoid tissues leads to systemic

inflammation, cytokine dysregulation, and immune cell activation, contributing to CD4 T-cell depletion, immune exhaustion, and disease progression.

2. **Lymphoid Tissue Fibrosis**: Persistent HIV replication and immune activation induce collagen deposition and fibrosis within lymphoid tissues, impairing immune cell trafficking, antigen presentation, and immune function, exacerbating immunodeficiency and complications.

Lymphatic System in HIV/AIDS Pathophysiology

Immunodeficiency and Opportunistic Infections

1. **CD4 T-Cell Depletion**: HIV selectively targets and depletes CD4 T-cells within lymphoid tissues, compromising adaptive immune responses and increasing susceptibility to opportunistic infections (e.g., Pneumocystis pneumonia, Mycobacterium avium complex).

2. **Impaired Immune Surveillance**: HIV-mediated damage to lymphoid tissues impairs immune surveillance and antigen presentation, reducing the ability to mount effective immune responses against opportunistic pathogens and malignancies.

HIV Dissemination and Systemic Effects

1. **Viral Spread**: Lymphatic vessels facilitate HIV dissemination from initial infection sites to systemic lymphoid tissues and bloodstream, promoting viral diversity, compartmentalization, and seeding of distant anatomical sites (e.g., central nervous system).

2. **Systemic Inflammation**: Dysregulated immune responses and chronic inflammation within lymphatic and systemic compartments contribute to HIV-associated comorbidities (e.g., cardiovascular disease, neurocognitive impairment) and accelerate HIV disease progression.

Diagnostic and Therapeutic Considerations

Lymph Node Examination

1. **Diagnostic Biopsy**: Lymph node biopsy and histopathological examination provide insights into HIV-associated lymphadenopathy, immune activation, granulomatous reactions, or opportunistic infections, guiding clinical management and therapeutic decisions.

Therapeutic Strategies

1. **ART Initiation**: Early initiation of ART suppresses HIV replication, preserves CD4 T-cells, and mitigates lymphoid tissue damage, reducing systemic viral load, immune activation, and the risk of opportunistic infections.
2. **Immunomodulatory Therapies**: Adjunctive therapies targeting immune dysregulation (e.g., anti-inflammatory agents, cytokine blockers) may alleviate chronic inflammation, preserve lymphoid tissue function, and improve immune reconstitution in HIV-infected individuals.

Conclusion

The lymphatic system is integral to immune surveillance, pathogen defense, and maintaining tissue homeostasis. In HIV/AIDS, HIV targets and disrupts lymphoid tissues, establishing viral reservoirs, inducing chronic immune activation, and compromising immune function. Understanding the intricate interactions between HIV and the lymphatic system informs diagnostic approaches, therapeutic strategies, and efforts towards achieving sustained viral suppression, immune reconstitution, and improving clinical outcomes in individuals living with HIV/AIDS. Continued research into lymphatic system dynamics and HIV pathogenesis is essential for advancing treatment innovations and addressing the global impact of HIV/AIDS.

Impact on Other Organs and Systems

Human Immunodeficiency Virus (HIV) infection has far-reaching consequences beyond the immune system, affecting multiple organs and systems throughout the body. Understanding the impact of HIV on these organs and systems is essential for comprehensive patient care, treatment strategies, and management of HIV/AIDS. This section explores the diverse manifestations of HIV-related complications in the central nervous system (CNS) and gastrointestinal (GI) system, highlighting pathophysiological mechanisms, clinical implications, diagnostic considerations, and therapeutic interventions.

Central Nervous System (CNS)

HIV can penetrate the blood-brain barrier (BBB) early in infection, leading to a spectrum of neurological complications collectively termed HIV-associated neurocognitive disorders (HAND). The CNS is particularly vulnerable to HIV due to its immunologically privileged status, viral tropism for glial cells and neurons, and persistent low-level viral replication despite effective antiretroviral therapy (ART).

HIV Neurotropism and CNS Entry

1. **BBB Penetration**: HIV-infected monocytes and lymphocytes cross the BBB during primary infection, establishing viral reservoirs within the CNS, including perivascular macrophages and microglia.
2. **Viral Tropism**: HIV exhibits neurotropism for microglial cells and astrocytes, leading to local viral replication, chronic inflammation, and neuronal damage within the CNS.

HIV-Associated Neurocognitive Disorders (HAND)

HAND encompasses a spectrum of cognitive, motor, and behavioral impairments, ranging from asymptomatic neurocognitive impairment (ANI) to mild neurocognitive disorder (MND) and HIV-associated dementia (HAD):

1. **Neurological Symptoms**: Cognitive deficits (e.g., memory loss, executive dysfunction), motor impairments (e.g., gait disturbances, weakness), and psychiatric symptoms (e.g., depression, apathy) manifest as HIV progresses.
2. **Pathophysiological Mechanisms**: HIV-induced neuroinflammation, oxidative stress, excitotoxicity, and synaptic dysfunction contribute to neuronal injury, white matter abnormalities, and neurodegeneration observed in HAND.

Diagnostic Approaches

1. **Neuroimaging**: Magnetic resonance imaging (MRI) and computed tomography (CT) scans detect HIV-related CNS abnormalities, including white matter lesions, brain atrophy, and opportunistic infections (e.g., toxoplasmosis, cryptococcosis).
2. **Cerebrospinal Fluid (CSF) Analysis**: CSF examination reveals elevated protein levels, pleocytosis, and detection of HIV RNA or DNA, aiding in the diagnosis of HIV-related CNS infections and neurocognitive impairment.

Therapeutic Strategies

1. **ART and CNS Penetration**: ART regimens with high CNS penetration effectiveness (CPE) reduce CNS viral load, control neuroinflammation, and improve neurocognitive function in HIV-infected individuals.
2. **Adjunctive Therapies**: Neuroprotective agents (e.g., memantine, minocycline) target neuroinflammatory pathways and neuronal injury mechanisms, potentially mitigating HAND progression and improving cognitive outcomes.

Gastrointestinal System

HIV profoundly impacts the gastrointestinal (GI) tract, involving structural changes, microbial alterations, immune dysregulation, and increased susceptibility to opportunistic infections and malignancies. The GI tract serves as a major reservoir for HIV replication and plays critical roles in immune homeostasis, nutrient absorption, and host-microbiome interactions.

HIV-Induced GI Tract Dysfunction

1. **Mucosal Immunity**: HIV targets gut-associated lymphoid tissue (GALT), leading to CD4 T-cell depletion, disruption of mucosal barrier integrity, and increased microbial translocation of gut commensal bacteria and microbial products into systemic circulation.
2. **Enteropathy and Malabsorption**: HIV-associated enteropathy manifests as chronic diarrhea, malabsorption syndromes (e.g., enteric pathogens, cryptosporidiosis), nutrient deficiencies, and weight loss, impairing nutritional status and overall health.

Microbial Dysbiosis and Opportunistic Infections

1. **Microbial Alterations**: HIV alters gut microbiota composition, reducing microbial diversity, and promoting dysbiosis associated with chronic inflammation, immune activation, and impaired host defense against opportunistic infections (e.g., cytomegalovirus, Mycobacterium avium complex).
2. **Opportunistic Infections**: GI tract infections (e.g., cytomegalovirus colitis, cryptosporidiosis) and malignancies (e.g., Kaposi's sarcoma, non-Hodgkin lymphoma) occur due to HIV-induced immune suppression and impaired mucosal immunity.

Gastrointestinal Symptoms and Complications

1. **Clinical Manifestations**: GI symptoms in HIV/AIDS include diarrhea, abdominal pain, nausea, vomiting,

dysphagia, and anorectal disorders, impacting quality of life and nutritional status.
2. **Structural Changes**: HIV-associated GI complications encompass mucosal ulcerations, villous atrophy, granulomatous inflammation, and opportunistic infections, complicating diagnostic evaluation and therapeutic management.

Diagnostic Considerations
1. **Endoscopic Evaluation**: Upper endoscopy and colonoscopy detect HIV-related GI abnormalities (e.g., ulcers, nodules, polyps) and facilitate tissue biopsy for histopathological diagnosis of opportunistic infections or malignancies.
2. **Stool Studies**: Microbiological analysis of stool samples identifies enteric pathogens (e.g., parasites, bacteria) responsible for HIV-associated diarrhea, guiding targeted antimicrobial therapy and supportive care interventions.

Therapeutic Strategies
1. **Antiretroviral Therapy (ART)**: Early initiation of ART suppresses HIV replication in the GI tract, preserves mucosal CD4 T-cell populations, restores gut barrier function, and reduces microbial translocation, improving GI tract health and immune reconstitution.
2. **Symptomatic Management**: Pharmacological interventions (e.g., anti-diarrheal agents, proton pump inhibitors) alleviate GI symptoms and complications, supporting nutritional absorption, and optimizing patient comfort and adherence to HIV treatment.

Conclusion

HIV infection exerts profound effects on multiple organ systems beyond the immune system, impacting the CNS and GI tract with diverse pathophysiological mechanisms, clinical manifestations, and therapeutic challenges. Understanding the complexities of HIV-related complications in the CNS and GI system informs diagnostic strategies, therapeutic interventions, and holistic patient care approaches aimed at mitigating disease progression, improving quality of life, and addressing the global impact of HIV/AIDS. Continued research into organ-specific manifestations, treatment innovations, and integrated healthcare models is essential for optimizing outcomes and achieving long-term management of HIV/AIDS worldwide.

CHAPTER 4: CLINICAL MANIFESTATIONS AND SYMPTOMS

Acute HIV Infection

Acute HIV infection represents the initial phase of Human Immunodeficiency Virus (HIV) infection, characterized by a transient yet critical period of viral replication, immune activation, and potential transmission. Understanding the dynamics of acute HIV infection is essential for early diagnosis, timely intervention, and effective prevention strategies. This section provides a comprehensive exploration of acute HIV infection, including epidemiology, clinical manifestations, immunological responses, diagnostic considerations, and implications for public health and clinical practice.

Epidemiology of Acute HIV Infection

Acute HIV infection is defined as the period immediately following HIV acquisition and initial viral exposure, encompassing the time from viral entry into host cells to the development of detectable HIV-specific antibodies. Key epidemiological aspects include:

- **Transmission Dynamics**: Acute HIV infection contributes significantly to HIV transmission dynamics due to high viral loads in blood and genital secretions during this early stage, posing increased risk of HIV acquisition for sexual partners and vertical transmission from mother to child.

- **Incidence Rates**: Incidence of acute HIV infection varies geographically and among populations with higher risk behaviors (e.g., men who have sex with men, intravenous drug users), underscoring the importance of targeted screening and prevention efforts.
- **Demographic Trends**: Young adults, particularly those engaging in high-risk behaviors or residing in regions with high HIV prevalence, are disproportionately affected by acute HIV infection, necessitating enhanced public health strategies for early detection and intervention.

Clinical Manifestations of Acute HIV Infection

Acute HIV infection is characterized by a spectrum of non-specific symptoms that resemble flu-like illness, occurring 2 to 4 weeks following HIV exposure. Common clinical manifestations include:

- **Fever**: Often the initial symptom, accompanied by night sweats and malaise.
- **Rash**: Maculopapular rash, typically involving the trunk and extremities.
- **Lymphadenopathy**: Generalized lymphadenopathy, particularly in cervical and inguinal regions.
- **Pharyngitis**: Sore throat and mucosal inflammation.
- **Other Symptoms**: Headache, myalgia, arthralgia, gastrointestinal disturbances (e.g., nausea, vomiting, diarrhea), and neurological symptoms (e.g., meningeal irritation).

These symptoms reflect systemic immune activation in response to viral replication and dissemination, preceding the establishment of viral reservoirs and immune suppression characteristic of chronic HIV infection.

Immunological Responses during Acute HIV Infection

Acute HIV infection triggers dynamic immunological responses aimed at controlling viral replication and limiting disease progression, involving innate and adaptive immune mechanisms:

- **Viral Replication**: Following viral entry into CD4 T-cells and other susceptible immune cells, HIV undergoes rapid replication in lymphoid tissues and systemic circulation, resulting in peak viremia within weeks of infection.
- **Innate Immune Activation**: Activation of innate immune cells (e.g., macrophages, dendritic cells) initiates pro-inflammatory cytokine release (e.g., TNF-alpha, IL-6), promoting immune activation and recruitment of adaptive immune responses.
- **Adaptive Immune Responses**: HIV-specific CD4 and CD8 T-cell responses develop during acute infection, targeting viral antigens presented by infected cells and contributing to initial control of viral replication and resolution of acute symptoms.
- **Humoral Immunity**: Production of HIV-specific antibodies, including non-neutralizing and neutralizing antibodies against viral envelope proteins (e.g., gp120, gp41), marks the transition from acute to chronic HIV infection and informs serological diagnosis.

Diagnostic Considerations for Acute HIV Infection

Early diagnosis of acute HIV infection is challenging due to non-specific clinical symptoms and the initial window period before detectable HIV antibodies. Diagnostic strategies include:

- **Serological Testing**: Initial detection of HIV-specific antibodies (IgM/IgG) using enzyme immunoassays (EIAs) and rapid diagnostic tests (RDTs) may yield false-negative results during the acute phase due to delayed seroconversion.

- **Nucleic Acid Testing (NAT)**: HIV RNA or DNA amplification assays (e.g., viral load testing, PCR) directly detect viral nucleic acids in blood or plasma, enabling early diagnosis of acute HIV infection during the window period before seroconversion.
- **Combined Testing Algorithms**: Sequential or parallel testing algorithms combining NAT and serological assays enhance diagnostic sensitivity and specificity for detecting acute HIV infection, facilitating early intervention and linkage to care.
- **Point-of-Care Testing**: Rapid HIV testing platforms capable of detecting viral antigens or antibodies within minutes enable immediate diagnosis and early treatment initiation in clinical and community settings.

Implications for Public Health and Clinical Practice

Effective management of acute HIV infection requires integrated approaches addressing clinical, epidemiological, and public health considerations:

- **Prevention Strategies**: Targeted HIV testing, risk reduction counseling, and pre-exposure prophylaxis (PrEP) promote early diagnosis, reduce onward transmission, and mitigate the impact of acute HIV infection on public health.
- **Early Intervention**: Prompt initiation of antiretroviral therapy (ART) during acute HIV infection suppresses viral replication, preserves immune function, and limits establishment of viral reservoirs, improving long-term clinical outcomes and reducing HIV transmission risk.
- **Screening Programs**: Expanded HIV screening programs incorporating routine testing, community outreach, and education efforts increase detection of acute HIV infection among high-risk populations and

facilitate timely linkage to comprehensive HIV care and support services.

- **Research and Surveillance**: Ongoing research into the pathogenesis of acute HIV infection, viral dynamics, immune responses, and novel therapeutic strategies informs evidence-based interventions and enhances global efforts towards achieving HIV prevention, treatment, and cure goals.

Conclusion

Acute HIV infection represents a critical phase of early viral dissemination, immune activation, and clinical manifestation preceding chronic HIV disease. Understanding the epidemiology, clinical features, immunological responses, diagnostic challenges, and public health implications of acute HIV infection is essential for optimizing screening strategies, early diagnosis, and timely intervention with antiretroviral therapy. Comprehensive approaches integrating clinical care, prevention efforts, and research initiatives are pivotal in mitigating the impact of acute HIV infection on individual health outcomes and global HIV/AIDS epidemic control efforts. Continued collaboration, innovation in diagnostic technologies, and community engagement are essential for advancing HIV prevention, treatment, and public health strategies worldwide.

Asymptomatic Phase of HIV Infection

The asymptomatic phase of Human Immunodeficiency Virus (HIV) infection, also known as chronic asymptomatic or clinical latency stage, represents a critical period characterized by persistent viral replication, immune modulation, and gradual immunological decline without overt clinical symptoms. Understanding the dynamics of the asymptomatic phase is crucial for early detection, management strategies, and optimizing long-term clinical outcomes in individuals living with HIV/AIDS. This section explores the epidemiology, immunopathogenesis, clinical course, diagnostic considerations, and therapeutic interventions during the asymptomatic phase of HIV infection.

Epidemiology of the Asymptomatic Phase

The asymptomatic phase of HIV infection typically follows the acute phase and precedes the onset of symptomatic HIV/AIDS. Key epidemiological aspects include:

- **Duration and Variability**: The duration of the asymptomatic phase varies widely among individuals, influenced by viral factors (e.g., HIV subtype, viral load set point), host immune responses, adherence to antiretroviral therapy (ART), and presence of co-infections or comorbidities.
- **Global Burden**: Globally, millions of individuals are in the asymptomatic phase of HIV infection, contributing to sustained transmission dynamics and public health challenges despite advancements in HIV prevention and treatment.
- **Demographic Trends**: Vulnerable populations, including men who have sex with men (MSM), transgender individuals, people who inject drugs (PWID), and marginalized communities, bear disproportionate burdens of undiagnosed and untreated HIV infection during the asymptomatic phase.

Immunopathogenesis of the Asymptomatic Phase

During the asymptomatic phase, HIV establishes persistent infection within target cells of the immune system, leading to dynamic interactions between viral replication, immune activation, and host immune responses:

- **Viral Reservoirs**: HIV persists in latent reservoirs within long-lived CD4 T-cells, macrophages, and other immune cells despite effective ART, contributing to viral persistence, intermittent viremia, and potential viral rebound upon treatment interruption.

- **Immune Modulation**: HIV-induced chronic immune activation and inflammation drive progressive CD4 T-cell depletion, immune exhaustion, and dysregulation of innate and adaptive immune responses, compromising host defense mechanisms against opportunistic infections and malignancies.
- **Host-Virus Interactions**: Viral factors (e.g., genetic diversity, mutation rates) and host immune factors (e.g., HLA haplotypes, immune escape mechanisms) influence disease progression rates, transmission dynamics, and response to therapeutic interventions during the asymptomatic phase.

Clinical Course and Natural History

The clinical course of HIV infection during the asymptomatic phase is characterized by a gradual decline in immune function, often asymptomatic or with mild, non-specific symptoms:

- **Clinical Stability**: Many individuals remain clinically stable during the asymptomatic phase, experiencing periods of undetectable viral load and preserved immune function with adherence to ART and regular medical monitoring.
- **Subclinical Symptoms**: Some individuals may experience non-specific symptoms such as fatigue, low-grade fever, lymphadenopathy, and intermittent viral shedding, reflecting ongoing viral replication and immune activation despite apparent clinical stability.
- **Long-Term Complications**: Prolonged untreated HIV infection during the asymptomatic phase increases the risk of developing HIV-associated comorbidities, including cardiovascular disease, neurocognitive impairment, renal dysfunction, and non-AIDS-defining cancers (e.g., lung cancer, anal cancer).

Diagnostic Considerations in the Asymptomatic Phase

Early detection of HIV infection during the asymptomatic phase is crucial for initiating timely ART, optimizing clinical outcomes, and reducing HIV transmission risk:

- **Routine HIV Testing**: Routine screening recommendations include HIV testing for all individuals aged 13-64 years as part of regular healthcare assessments, with targeted testing strategies for high-risk populations and settings with elevated HIV prevalence.
- **Serological Testing**: Detection of HIV-specific antibodies (IgM/IgG) using enzyme immunoassays (EIAs) and rapid diagnostic tests (RDTs) remains the cornerstone of serological HIV testing algorithms, indicating recent or past HIV exposure.
- **Viral Load Monitoring**: Quantitative measurement of HIV RNA levels using nucleic acid testing (NAT) assesses viral replication dynamics, guides treatment decisions, and monitors response to ART during the asymptomatic phase.
- **CD4 T-Cell Count**: Immunological monitoring through CD4 T-cell enumeration provides insights into immune status, predicts the risk of opportunistic infections, and informs timing of ART initiation and preventative interventions.

Therapeutic Interventions and Management Strategies

Effective management of HIV infection during the asymptomatic phase focuses on early ART initiation, adherence to treatment guidelines, and comprehensive healthcare approaches:

- **Antiretroviral Therapy (ART)**: Early initiation of ART suppresses viral replication, preserves immune function, reduces the risk of HIV-associated complications, and enhances long-term clinical outcomes in individuals living with HIV/AIDS.

- **Treatment Guidelines**: Current treatment guidelines recommend ART initiation regardless of CD4 T-cell count or clinical symptoms during the asymptomatic phase to achieve sustained viral suppression, immune reconstitution, and optimize overall health.
- **Monitoring and Adherence**: Regular medical monitoring, adherence to ART regimens, management of treatment-related side effects, and supportive care interventions promote treatment adherence and improve quality of life for individuals living with HIV/AIDS.

Public Health and Policy Implications

Addressing the challenges of HIV infection during the asymptomatic phase requires integrated approaches encompassing public health initiatives, policy advocacy, and community engagement:

- **HIV Prevention**: Combination prevention strategies, including HIV testing, condom use, harm reduction programs for PWID, pre-exposure prophylaxis (PrEP), and behavioral interventions, reduce HIV transmission risk and enhance early diagnosis during the asymptomatic phase.
- **Healthcare Infrastructure**: Strengthening healthcare systems, expanding access to HIV testing and treatment services, integrating HIV care with primary healthcare settings, and reducing disparities in healthcare access promote equitable HIV/AIDS care and support.
- **Research and Innovation**: Continued research into HIV pathogenesis, viral reservoirs, immune responses, and novel therapeutic approaches advances scientific understanding, informs evidence-based interventions, and drives progress towards achieving global HIV/AIDS goals.

Conclusion

The asymptomatic phase of HIV infection represents a pivotal stage characterized by persistent viral replication, immune modulation, and gradual immunological decline without overt clinical symptoms. Understanding the epidemiology, immunopathogenesis, clinical course, diagnostic considerations, therapeutic interventions, and public health implications during the asymptomatic phase is essential for optimizing HIV/AIDS management strategies, enhancing early detection, promoting treatment adherence, and improving long-term clinical outcomes for individuals living with HIV/AIDS worldwide. Comprehensive approaches integrating medical advances, public health initiatives, and community empowerment efforts are instrumental in achieving sustained viral suppression, reducing HIV transmission, and ultimately, advancing towards global HIV/AIDS epidemic control and eradication goals.

Asymptomatic Phase of HIV Infection

The asymptomatic phase of Human Immunodeficiency Virus (HIV) infection, often referred to as clinical latency, is a critical period characterized by stable viral replication, relative immune quiescence, and absence of overt clinical symptoms associated with HIV/AIDS. Despite the absence of noticeable symptoms, HIV continues to replicate actively within the host, leading to gradual immune system deterioration and potential long-term complications if left untreated. This phase plays a crucial role in the natural history of HIV infection, influencing disease progression, treatment outcomes, and public health strategies. This section provides a comprehensive exploration of the asymptomatic phase, encompassing epidemiology, immunopathogenesis, clinical aspects, diagnostic considerations, management strategies, and public health implications.

Epidemiology of the Asymptomatic Phase

The asymptomatic phase of HIV infection follows the acute phase and may last for several years or even decades before progressing to symptomatic HIV/AIDS. Understanding the epidemiological patterns and demographic factors associated with this phase is essential:

- **Duration and Variability**: The duration of the asymptomatic phase varies widely among individuals and depends on multiple factors, including viral factors (such as subtype and replication rate), host immune responses, genetic factors, and adherence to antiretroviral therapy (ART).
- **Global Burden**: Globally, millions of individuals are in the asymptomatic phase of HIV infection, contributing to ongoing transmission dynamics and public health challenges. In some regions, delayed diagnosis and treatment initiation prolong the asymptomatic phase, potentially increasing the risk of onward transmission.
- **Demographic Trends**: Vulnerable populations, including men who have sex with men (MSM), transgender individuals, people who inject drugs (PWID), and marginalized communities, may experience disparities in accessing HIV testing, prevention services, and timely ART initiation during the asymptomatic phase.

Immunopathogenesis of the Asymptomatic Phase

During the asymptomatic phase, HIV establishes a delicate equilibrium within the host immune system, characterized by ongoing viral replication, immune activation, and gradual immune dysfunction:

- **Viral Reservoirs**: HIV persists primarily in long-lived CD4+ T-cells and macrophages, forming latent reservoirs that are not fully eradicated by current ART regimens. These reservoirs allow for intermittent viral replication and occasional viral escape despite effective suppression of plasma viremia.

- **Immune Modulation**: Chronic HIV infection leads to persistent immune activation and inflammation, characterized by elevated levels of pro-inflammatory cytokines (such as TNF-alpha, IL-6) and markers of immune activation (e.g., CD38 and HLA-DR expression on T-cells). This immune activation accelerates CD4+ T-cell turnover and contributes to immune exhaustion over time.
- **Host-Virus Interactions**: The interplay between host immune responses and viral factors influences disease progression rates, viral set point (the stable level of viremia reached after acute infection), and the risk of developing opportunistic infections and non-AIDS-defining complications during the asymptomatic phase.

Clinical Course and Natural History

The clinical course of HIV infection during the asymptomatic phase is typically characterized by stability in clinical parameters, absence of significant symptoms, and preservation of overall health:

- **Clinical Stability**: Many individuals in the asymptomatic phase maintain stable CD4+ T-cell counts and undetectable or low-level viremia with adherence to ART. This period is often marked by a lack of specific symptoms related to HIV/AIDS, although some individuals may experience non-specific symptoms such as fatigue or mild lymphadenopathy.
- **Subclinical Manifestations**: Despite the absence of clinical symptoms, ongoing immune activation and viral replication may lead to subclinical manifestations, including persistent low-level

viremia, immune dysregulation, and subtle changes in inflammatory markers and immune cell subsets.
- **Long-Term Complications**: Prolonged untreated HIV infection during the asymptomatic phase increases the risk of developing HIV-associated comorbidities, including cardiovascular disease, neurocognitive impairment, renal dysfunction, and certain malignancies (such as lymphomas and cancers of the cervix, lung, and liver).

Diagnostic Considerations in the Asymptomatic Phase

Early detection of HIV infection during the asymptomatic phase is critical for timely initiation of ART, prevention of disease progression, and reduction of HIV transmission risk:

- **HIV Testing Strategies**: Routine HIV testing is recommended for all individuals aged 13-64 years as part of comprehensive healthcare assessments. HIV testing algorithms typically include initial screening with HIV antibody tests (e.g., ELISA) followed by confirmatory tests (e.g., Western blot) to diagnose HIV infection.
- **Viral Load Monitoring**: Quantitative measurement of HIV RNA levels in plasma or blood provides valuable information on viral replication dynamics, informs treatment decisions, and monitors the effectiveness of ART during the asymptomatic phase.
- **CD4+ T-Cell Count**: Measurement of CD4+ T-cell counts through flow cytometry or other methods assesses immune status, predicts the risk of opportunistic infections, and guides the timing of ART initiation in asymptomatic individuals with declining CD4+ T-cell counts.
- **Serological Markers**: Detection of HIV-specific antibodies (IgM/IgG) and other serological markers (e.g., p24 antigen) may indicate recent HIV exposure or

ongoing viral replication, facilitating early diagnosis and intervention.

Therapeutic Interventions and Management Strategies

Management of HIV infection during the asymptomatic phase focuses on early initiation of ART, adherence to treatment guidelines, monitoring of clinical and immunological parameters, and comprehensive healthcare approaches:

- **Antiretroviral Therapy (ART)**: Early initiation of ART is recommended for all individuals diagnosed with HIV infection, regardless of CD4+ T-cell count or clinical symptoms. ART suppresses viral replication, preserves immune function, reduces the risk of HIV-associated complications, and enhances long-term clinical outcomes.

- **Treatment Guidelines**: Current treatment guidelines emphasize the importance of ART adherence, regular monitoring of viral load and CD4+ T-cell counts, management of treatment-related side effects, and screening for comorbidities (such as hepatitis B and C co-infections) during the asymptomatic phase.

- **Patient Education and Support**: Counseling on ART adherence, HIV transmission prevention strategies (such as condom use and harm reduction), and lifestyle modifications (including smoking cessation and vaccination against opportunistic infections) promotes patient empowerment and improves overall health outcomes.

Public Health and Policy Implications

Addressing the challenges of HIV infection during the asymptomatic phase requires coordinated efforts across public health sectors, policy advocacy, and community engagement:

- **HIV Prevention**: Comprehensive HIV prevention strategies include scaling up HIV testing and counseling services, promoting access to PrEP (pre-exposure prophylaxis) for high-risk individuals, and implementing harm reduction programs for PWID to reduce HIV transmission risk.

- **Healthcare Infrastructure**: Strengthening healthcare systems through integration of HIV care with primary healthcare settings, expanding access to ART and diagnostic technologies, and reducing disparities in healthcare access promotes equitable HIV/AIDS care and support.
- **Research and Innovation**: Continued research into HIV pathogenesis, viral reservoir dynamics, immune responses, and novel therapeutic approaches drives scientific advancements, informs evidence-based interventions, and supports global efforts towards achieving HIV/AIDS epidemic control and eradication goals.

Conclusion

The asymptomatic phase of HIV infection represents a pivotal period characterized by persistent viral replication, immune modulation, and gradual immune dysfunction in the absence of overt clinical symptoms. Understanding the epidemiology, immunopathogenesis, clinical course, diagnostic considerations, therapeutic interventions, and public health implications during the asymptomatic phase is essential for optimizing HIV/AIDS management strategies, enhancing early detection, promoting treatment adherence, and improving long-term clinical outcomes for individuals living with HIV/AIDS worldwide. Comprehensive approaches integrating medical advances, public health initiatives, and community empowerment efforts are instrumental in achieving sustained viral suppression, reducing HIV transmission, and advancing towards global HIV/AIDS epidemic control and eradication goals.

Early Symptoms and Seroconversion in HIV Infection

Early symptoms and seroconversion represent critical phases in the progression of Human Immunodeficiency Virus (HIV) infection, marking the transition from acute to chronic stages. Understanding these phases is essential for timely diagnosis, initiation of treatment, and management of HIV/AIDS. This section provides a comprehensive exploration of early symptoms, seroconversion dynamics, clinical manifestations, diagnostic considerations, and implications for public health and clinical practice.

Early Symptoms of HIV Infection

Early symptoms of HIV infection typically manifest during the acute phase, occurring 2 to 4 weeks following initial exposure to the virus. These symptoms, often resembling flu-like illness, result from rapid viral replication and immune activation:

- **Fever**: Persistent or intermittent fever, often accompanied by night sweats and chills.
- **Lymphadenopathy**: Generalized lymphadenopathy with painless swelling of lymph nodes, particularly in the cervical, axillary, and inguinal regions.
- **Rash**: Maculopapular rash, commonly affecting the trunk, face, and extremities.
- **Pharyngitis**: Sore throat and inflammation of the pharyngeal mucosa.
- **Fatigue**: Persistent fatigue and malaise, contributing to overall discomfort.

These early symptoms reflect systemic immune activation and inflammatory responses to HIV replication within the host, preceding the development of detectable HIV-specific antibodies (seroconversion) and onset of chronic asymptomatic infection.

Dynamics of Seroconversion

Seroconversion refers to the development of detectable HIV-specific antibodies in blood or serum, typically occurring 2 to 8 weeks following initial HIV exposure. The process of seroconversion is characterized by distinct immunological and virological dynamics:

- **Window Period**: The window period represents the interval between HIV acquisition and the appearance of detectable HIV antibodies in blood, during which standard antibody tests (e.g., ELISA) may yield false-negative results despite ongoing viral replication and potential transmission risk.
- **Antibody Production**: Following HIV exposure, host immune cells recognize viral antigens (e.g., gp120, gp41) and initiate production of HIV-specific antibodies, including both non-neutralizing and neutralizing antibodies targeting different regions of the viral envelope.
- **Diagnostic Markers**: Laboratory diagnosis of HIV infection during seroconversion relies on serial testing algorithms, including initial screening with antibody tests (e.g., ELISA) followed by confirmatory tests (e.g., Western blot or nucleic acid testing) to distinguish between acute HIV infection and false-positive results.

Clinical Manifestations during Early HIV Infection

Early HIV infection is characterized by a spectrum of clinical manifestations, varying in severity and duration among affected individuals:

- **Acute Retroviral Syndrome**: Acute retroviral syndrome (ARS) encompasses the constellation of symptoms associated with early HIV infection, typically lasting for 1 to 2 weeks. In addition to fever, lymphadenopathy, rash, and pharyngitis, individuals may experience neurological symptoms (e.g., headache, meningismus), gastrointestinal

disturbances (e.g., nausea, vomiting, diarrhea), myalgia, and arthralgia.
- **Variability in Symptoms**: The clinical presentation of early HIV infection can vary widely among individuals, influenced by viral factors (e.g., HIV subtype, viral load), host immune responses, and pre-existing health conditions. Some individuals may present with mild or atypical symptoms, leading to under-recognition and delayed diagnosis.
- **Progression to Chronic Infection**: In untreated individuals, early HIV infection progresses to chronic asymptomatic infection following resolution of acute symptoms and establishment of viral reservoirs within immune cells, contributing to persistent viral replication and immune dysfunction.

Diagnostic Considerations for Early HIV Infection

Early diagnosis of HIV infection during the acute phase and seroconversion is crucial for timely initiation of antiretroviral therapy (ART), reducing HIV transmission risk, and improving long-term clinical outcomes:

- **Screening Strategies**: Routine HIV screening is recommended for all individuals aged 13-64 years as part of comprehensive healthcare assessments. Targeted screening strategies for high-risk populations (e.g., MSM, PWID) and individuals with potential HIV exposure optimize early detection and linkage to HIV care services.
- **Diagnostic Testing**: Laboratory diagnosis of early HIV infection involves sequential testing algorithms, beginning with HIV antibody tests (e.g., ELISA) and supplemented by confirmatory tests (e.g., Western blot or nucleic acid testing) to differentiate between acute HIV infection, recent seroconversion, and false-positive results.

- **Nucleic Acid Testing (NAT)**: Detection of HIV RNA or DNA through NAT provides early diagnosis of acute HIV infection during the window period before seroconversion, informing treatment decisions and reducing the risk of undiagnosed HIV transmission.
- **Point-of-Care Testing**: Rapid HIV tests (e.g., rapid antibody tests, point-of-care NAT) enable immediate diagnosis in clinical and community settings, facilitating early linkage to HIV care and support services.

Public Health and Clinical Implications

Effective management of early symptoms and seroconversion in HIV infection requires coordinated efforts across public health sectors, healthcare providers, and community organizations:

- **Treatment Initiation**: Early initiation of ART during acute HIV infection suppresses viral replication, preserves immune function, and reduces the risk of HIV-associated complications, enhancing long-term clinical outcomes and quality of life.
- **Prevention Strategies**: Combination HIV prevention strategies, including HIV testing, PrEP for high-risk individuals, condom use, and harm reduction programs, reduce HIV transmission risk and promote early diagnosis of acute infection and seroconversion.
- **Healthcare Infrastructure**: Strengthening healthcare systems through integration of HIV testing, treatment, and supportive services promotes timely diagnosis, retention in care, and adherence to ART among individuals with early HIV infection.
- **Research and Innovation**: Continued research into the immunological mechanisms of seroconversion, viral dynamics, host-virus interactions, and novel therapeutic interventions informs evidence-based approaches and supports global efforts towards HIV/

AIDS epidemic control and eradication.

Conclusion

Early symptoms and seroconversion represent pivotal phases in the natural history of HIV infection, marking the transition from acute to chronic stages and influencing disease progression, treatment outcomes, and public health strategies. Understanding the dynamics of early HIV infection, including clinical manifestations, seroconversion dynamics, diagnostic considerations, and implications for public health and clinical practice, is essential for optimizing HIV/AIDS management strategies, enhancing early detection, promoting treatment adherence, and reducing HIV transmission worldwide. Comprehensive approaches integrating medical advancements, public health initiatives, and community engagement efforts are instrumental in achieving sustained viral suppression, improving health outcomes, and advancing towards global HIV/AIDS epidemic control and eradication goals.

Advanced HIV Infection and AIDS

Advanced Human Immunodeficiency Virus (HIV) infection represents a critical stage characterized by profound immune suppression, increased susceptibility to opportunistic infections, AIDS-defining malignancies, and neurological complications. This section provides a comprehensive exploration of advanced HIV infection and acquired immunodeficiency syndrome (AIDS), including epidemiology, clinical manifestations, diagnostic considerations, management strategies, and public health implications.

Epidemiology of Advanced HIV Infection and AIDS

Advanced HIV infection and AIDS encompass the clinical spectrum of HIV/AIDS characterized by severe immune compromise and increased vulnerability to opportunistic infections and AIDS-defining conditions:

- **Global Burden**: Despite advancements in HIV treatment and prevention, millions of individuals worldwide progress to advanced HIV infection and AIDS, particularly in resource-limited settings with barriers to healthcare access, late diagnosis, and treatment initiation.
- **Demographic Trends**: Vulnerable populations, including socioeconomically disadvantaged individuals, marginalized communities, and those with limited access to HIV care services, experience disproportionate burdens of advanced HIV infection and AIDS-related morbidity and mortality.
- **Impact of ART**: Effective antiretroviral therapy (ART) has significantly reduced the incidence of advanced HIV infection and AIDS-related complications in high-income countries, highlighting the importance of early diagnosis, timely ART initiation, and sustained viral suppression in improving clinical outcomes.

Clinical Manifestations of Advanced HIV Infection and AIDS

Advanced HIV infection and AIDS are characterized by a spectrum of clinical manifestations, including opportunistic infections, AIDS-defining malignancies, and neurological complications:

Opportunistic Infections

Opportunistic infections (OIs) are infections caused by pathogens that typically do not cause disease in individuals with intact immune function but can result in severe illness in immunocompromised individuals:

- **Fungal Infections**: Pneumocystis jirovecii pneumonia (PCP), candidiasis (oral/esophageal), cryptococcal meningitis.
- **Bacterial Infections**: Mycobacterium tuberculosis (TB), Mycobacterium avium complex (MAC), bacterial pneumonia.

- **Viral Infections**: Cytomegalovirus (CMV) retinitis, herpes simplex virus (HSV) infection, varicella-zoster virus (VZV) infection.
- **Parasitic Infections**: Toxoplasmosis, Cryptosporidiosis, Isosporiasis.

AIDS-Defining Cancers

AIDS-defining cancers are malignancies that occur at increased frequencies in individuals with advanced HIV infection and AIDS, often indicating severe immunosuppression:

- **Kaposi's Sarcoma**: HHV-8-associated vascular tumor, characterized by cutaneous lesions, mucosal involvement, and visceral manifestations (e.g., pulmonary and gastrointestinal involvement).
- **Non-Hodgkin Lymphoma**: B-cell lymphomas, including diffuse large B-cell lymphoma and Burkitt lymphoma, associated with Epstein-Barr virus (EBV) and other oncogenic viruses.
- **Cervical Cancer**: Increased incidence of human papillomavirus (HPV)-related cervical intraepithelial neoplasia (CIN) and invasive cervical carcinoma in HIV-positive individuals.

Neurological Complications

Neurological complications in advanced HIV infection and AIDS encompass a spectrum of disorders affecting the central and peripheral nervous systems:

- **HIV-Associated Neurocognitive Disorders (HAND)**: Cognitive impairment ranging from mild neurocognitive disorder (MND) to HIV-associated dementia (HAD), characterized by cognitive decline, motor dysfunction, and behavioral changes.
- **Cryptococcal Meningitis**: Fungal infection of the meninges caused by Cryptococcus neoformans, presenting with headache, fever, altered mental status,

and signs of meningeal irritation.
- **Progressive Multifocal Leukoencephalopathy (PML)**: Opportunistic viral infection of the central nervous system caused by JC virus, leading to demyelination, motor deficits, cognitive impairment, and neurological decline.
- **Peripheral Neuropathy**: Distal symmetric polyneuropathy (DSPN), characterized by sensory loss, paresthesias, and motor weakness, attributed to HIV-related immune dysfunction and toxic effects of ART.

Diagnostic Considerations for Advanced HIV Infection and AIDS

Diagnosis and management of advanced HIV infection and AIDS require comprehensive clinical evaluation, laboratory testing, and targeted diagnostic interventions:

- **Immunological Monitoring**: Monitoring CD4+ T-cell counts and HIV RNA levels (viral load) guides disease staging, informs treatment decisions, and predicts the risk of opportunistic infections and AIDS-related complications.
- **Diagnostic Testing**: Diagnostic workup includes screening for opportunistic infections (e.g., blood cultures, sputum analysis, cerebrospinal fluid examination), serological testing for AIDS-defining cancers (e.g., HHV-8 serology, HPV testing), and neuroimaging studies (e.g., MRI) for neurological complications.
- **Histopathological Examination**: Tissue biopsy and histopathological examination confirm the diagnosis of AIDS-defining cancers (e.g., Kaposi's sarcoma, non-Hodgkin lymphoma) and guide therapeutic interventions, including chemotherapy, radiation therapy, and targeted antiviral treatments.

Management Strategies for Advanced HIV Infection and AIDS

Effective management of advanced HIV infection and AIDS focuses on multidisciplinary approaches, including antiretroviral therapy (ART), treatment of opportunistic infections, supportive care, and preventive interventions:

- **Antiretroviral Therapy (ART)**: Immediate initiation of ART is recommended for all individuals diagnosed with advanced HIV infection and AIDS to suppress viral replication, restore immune function, and reduce the risk of AIDS-related complications.
- **Treatment of Opportunistic Infections**: Prompt diagnosis and treatment of opportunistic infections with antimicrobial agents (e.g., antibiotics, antifungals, antivirals) improve clinical outcomes, reduce morbidity, and prevent disease progression.
- **Symptom Management**: Symptomatic management addresses pain, fatigue, gastrointestinal symptoms, and neurological deficits associated with advanced HIV infection and AIDS, enhancing quality of life and promoting adherence to therapeutic regimens.
- **Psychosocial Support**: Comprehensive care includes psychosocial support, counseling services, nutritional support, and adherence counseling to address psychosocial factors, treatment adherence barriers, and stigma associated with HIV/AIDS.

Public Health and Clinical Implications

Addressing the challenges of advanced HIV infection and AIDS requires integrated approaches across public health sectors, healthcare providers, and community organizations:

- **Prevention Strategies**: Combination prevention strategies, including HIV testing, early diagnosis, PrEP for high-risk individuals, condom use, and harm reduction programs, reduce HIV transmission risk and mitigate the impact of advanced HIV infection and AIDS on affected populations.

- **Healthcare Infrastructure**: Strengthening healthcare systems through capacity-building initiatives, training healthcare providers in HIV/AIDS care and management, and expanding access to ART and diagnostic technologies promote timely diagnosis, treatment initiation, and retention in HIV care.
- **Research and Innovation**: Continued research into novel therapeutic approaches, immune-based interventions, HIV reservoir eradication strategies, and vaccines informs evidence-based practices, enhances clinical outcomes, and supports global efforts towards HIV/AIDS epidemic control and eradication.

Conclusion

Advanced HIV infection and acquired immunodeficiency syndrome (AIDS) represent critical stages in the natural history of HIV/AIDS, characterized by severe immune compromise, increased susceptibility to opportunistic infections, AIDS-defining malignancies, and neurological complications. Understanding the epidemiology, clinical manifestations, diagnostic considerations, management strategies, and public health implications of advanced HIV infection and AIDS is essential for optimizing HIV/AIDS care, improving clinical outcomes, and reducing HIV transmission worldwide. Comprehensive approaches integrating medical advancements, public health interventions, and community engagement efforts are crucial in achieving sustained viral suppression, enhancing quality of life for individuals living with HIV/AIDS, and advancing towards global HIV/AIDS epidemic control and eradication goals.

CHAPTER 5: DIAGNOSTIC METHODS

Screening Tests for HIV

Screening for Human Immunodeficiency Virus (HIV) infection is a cornerstone of public health strategies aimed at early detection, timely intervention, and reducing HIV transmission. This section explores the principles, methodologies, advancements, and clinical implications of screening tests for HIV, encompassing laboratory-based assays, point-of-care tests, diagnostic algorithms, screening strategies, and global health considerations.

Introduction to HIV Screening

HIV screening refers to the systematic process of identifying individuals at risk of HIV infection through diagnostic testing, regardless of clinical symptoms or perceived risk factors. Screening aims to detect HIV infection early, facilitate linkage to care and treatment services, prevent HIV transmission, and improve long-term health outcomes for affected individuals. Effective screening programs are essential components of comprehensive HIV prevention and control efforts worldwide.

Principles of HIV Screening Tests

HIV screening tests are designed to detect either HIV-specific antibodies or viral antigens (or nucleic acids) in biological specimens, indicating current or recent HIV infection. Key principles guiding the development and implementation of HIV

screening tests include:
- **Sensitivity and Specificity**: Sensitivity refers to the ability of a test to correctly identify individuals with HIV infection (true positive rate), while specificity denotes the ability to correctly identify individuals without HIV infection (true negative rate). High sensitivity and specificity minimize false-positive and false-negative results, ensuring accurate diagnosis and subsequent management decisions.
- **Window Period**: The window period represents the interval between HIV acquisition and the detectability of HIV-specific markers (e.g., antibodies, antigens) in blood or serum. Advanced screening tests aim to shorten the window period through enhanced assay sensitivity and detection of early HIV infection, reducing missed diagnoses during the acute phase.
- **Laboratory Standards**: HIV screening tests adhere to rigorous quality assurance standards, including proficiency testing, external quality assessment programs, and adherence to regulatory guidelines (e.g., FDA approval, CE marking). Compliance with these standards ensures the reliability, reproducibility, and accuracy of screening test results across different healthcare settings.

Types of HIV Screening Tests

HIV screening tests encompass a range of laboratory-based assays and point-of-care (POC) tests designed to detect HIV-specific markers in various biological specimens, including blood, plasma, serum, oral fluid, and urine. Commonly used screening tests include:

1. Laboratory-Based Assays
- **Enzyme-Linked Immunosorbent Assay (ELISA)**: ELISA detects HIV-specific antibodies (IgM/IgG) or antigens (e.g., p24 antigen) in serum or

plasma samples. Positive results are confirmed by supplementary testing (e.g., Western blot, immunofluorescence assay) to distinguish between acute HIV infection, chronic infection, and false-positive results.

- **Chemiluminescent Immunoassay (CLIA)**: CLIA combines chemiluminescent substrates with antibody-antigen interactions for sensitive detection of HIV-specific antibodies and antigens. CLIA assays offer automated platforms, high throughput, and enhanced detection limits compared to traditional ELISA methods.
- **Nucleic Acid Testing (NAT)**: NAT detects HIV RNA or DNA in blood or plasma samples, providing early diagnosis during the window period before seroconversion. NAT is used for diagnostic confirmation in acute HIV infection, monitoring viral load in individuals on ART, and screening blood donations to prevent transfusion-transmitted HIV infection.

2. **Point-of-Care (POC) Tests**

- **Rapid Antibody Tests**: POC rapid tests detect HIV-specific antibodies (IgM/IgG) in whole blood, plasma, or oral fluid within minutes, facilitating immediate diagnosis and linkage to care in clinical and community settings. Rapid tests are user-friendly, require minimal training, and support decentralized HIV testing initiatives.
- **Rapid Antigen Tests**: POC rapid antigen tests detect HIV-specific antigens (e.g., p24 antigen) in blood or plasma samples, providing early detection of acute HIV infection during the window period. Antigen tests are integrated with antibody tests in dual-test algorithms for comprehensive HIV screening and diagnosis.

- **Combined Antigen-Antibody Tests**: Dual-test POC assays simultaneously detect HIV-specific antibodies and antigens in a single test device, enhancing diagnostic accuracy, shortening the window period, and facilitating immediate decision-making regarding HIV status and follow-up care.

Diagnostic Algorithms for HIV Screening

Diagnostic algorithms for HIV screening integrate sequential testing strategies, incorporating initial screening assays followed by confirmatory tests to optimize diagnostic accuracy and minimize false-positive and false-negative results:

- **Screening Phase**: Initial screening involves testing for HIV-specific markers (e.g., antibodies, antigens) using sensitive and specific assays (e.g., rapid antibody tests, ELISA). Reactive (positive) screening results require confirmation through supplementary testing to differentiate acute HIV infection from false-positive results.
- **Confirmatory Phase**: Confirmatory testing confirms the presence of HIV infection through supplementary assays (e.g., Western blot, line immunoassay) that detect specific HIV antibodies against multiple viral antigens. Positive results on confirmatory testing establish a definitive diagnosis of HIV infection, guiding subsequent clinical management and treatment decisions.

Screening Strategies and Public Health Considerations

Effective HIV screening strategies encompass targeted testing approaches, routine screening initiatives, and community-based outreach programs to reach populations at increased risk of HIV infection:

- **Targeted Testing**: Targeted screening focuses on high-risk populations, including men who have sex with men (MSM), people who inject drugs

(PWID), transgender individuals, sex workers, and individuals from HIV-endemic regions. Tailored testing approaches improve HIV case detection, facilitate early diagnosis, and reduce HIV transmission within priority populations.

- **Routine Screening**: Routine HIV screening is recommended for all individuals aged 13-64 years as part of routine healthcare assessments, irrespective of perceived risk factors. Routine screening initiatives increase HIV testing uptake, promote early diagnosis, and support timely initiation of ART to improve clinical outcomes and reduce HIV transmission at the population level.
- **Community-Based Testing**: Community-based HIV testing programs engage community health workers, peer educators, and outreach teams to provide accessible, stigma-free HIV testing services in diverse settings (e.g., clinics, mobile units, community centers). Community-based testing initiatives promote HIV awareness, encourage regular testing, and enhance linkage to care for HIV-positive individuals.

Clinical Implications and Management Strategies

HIV screening plays a pivotal role in clinical practice, public health policy, and HIV/AIDS management strategies:

- **Early Diagnosis**: Early detection of HIV infection through screening facilitates prompt initiation of ART, preserves immune function, and reduces the risk of AIDS-related complications and mortality.
- **Linkage to Care**: Positive screening results require timely linkage to HIV care services, including comprehensive clinical evaluation, initiation of ART, monitoring of viral load and CD4+ T-cell counts, and management of co-occurring infections and

comorbidities.
- **Prevention of Transmission**: Screening identifies individuals with undiagnosed HIV infection, enabling targeted prevention strategies (e.g., PrEP for HIV-negative individuals at high risk) and behavioral interventions to reduce HIV transmission within communities.

Future Directions and Innovations

Future advancements in HIV screening technologies and strategies aim to enhance diagnostic accuracy, expand access to testing services, and address evolving challenges in global HIV/AIDS control:

- **Next-Generation Assays**: Continued development of next-generation assays (e.g., multiplex serological assays, digital immunoassays) improves assay sensitivity, specificity, and throughput for comprehensive HIV screening and diagnosis.
- **Innovative Testing Platforms**: Integration of novel testing platforms (e.g., smartphone-based diagnostics, microfluidic devices) supports decentralized testing, enhances accessibility to HIV testing services in resource-limited settings, and promotes community-based HIV prevention and care initiatives.
- **Public Health Integration**: Integration of HIV screening with broader public health initiatives (e.g., TB control programs, maternal and child health services) strengthens healthcare systems, optimizes resource allocation, and advances progress towards achieving global HIV/AIDS epidemic control and elimination goals.

Conclusion

HIV screening tests are pivotal tools in the global response to HIV/AIDS, facilitating early detection, linkage to care, and prevention strategies to reduce HIV transmission and improve clinical outcomes. Understanding the principles, methodologies, advancements, diagnostic algorithms, screening strategies, and public health implications of HIV screening is essential for healthcare providers, policymakers, and community stakeholders involved in HIV/AIDS prevention, treatment, and care. Comprehensive approaches integrating medical innovations, public health initiatives, and community engagement efforts are critical in achieving universal access to HIV testing, enhancing HIV/AIDS management strategies, and advancing towards global HIV/AIDS epidemic control and elimination goals.

Confirmatory Tests and Viral Load Measurement in HIV Diagnosis

Confirmatory tests and viral load measurement play integral roles in the accurate diagnosis, clinical management, and monitoring of Human Immunodeficiency Virus (HIV) infection. This section explores the principles, methodologies, clinical implications, and advancements in confirmatory testing and viral load measurement, highlighting their significance in HIV/AIDS care.

Introduction to Confirmatory Tests in HIV Diagnosis

Confirmatory tests are essential components of HIV diagnostic algorithms, following initial screening to differentiate between true-positive HIV infection and false-positive results. These tests confirm the presence of HIV-specific markers (e.g., antibodies, antigens) and guide subsequent clinical management decisions, including initiation of antiretroviral therapy (ART) and monitoring of disease progression.

Principles of Confirmatory Tests

Confirmatory tests for HIV diagnosis adhere to key principles to ensure accuracy, reliability, and clinical utility:

- **Specificity**: Confirmatory tests are highly specific,

detecting HIV-specific antibodies against multiple viral antigens (e.g., gp160, gp120, p24) or viral nucleic acids (e.g., HIV RNA or DNA) to minimize false-positive results and confirm true HIV infection.
- **Sensitivity**: Confirmatory tests are sensitive, detecting HIV-specific markers at low concentrations in blood or serum samples to ensure accurate diagnosis during different stages of HIV infection, including acute and chronic phases.
- **Validation**: Validation of confirmatory tests involves rigorous quality control measures, proficiency testing, and adherence to regulatory guidelines (e.g., FDA approval, CE marking) to maintain assay performance and reliability across diverse healthcare settings.

Types of Confirmatory Tests

Confirmatory tests for HIV diagnosis encompass laboratory-based assays and molecular techniques designed to confirm the presence of HIV-specific markers and distinguish between acute HIV infection, chronic infection, and false-positive results:

1. Western Blot Assay
- **Principle**: Western blot assay detects HIV-specific antibodies (IgM/IgG) against multiple viral antigens (e.g., gp160, gp120, p24) in serum or plasma samples.
- **Procedure**: Serum or plasma proteins are separated by gel electrophoresis, transferred to a membrane, and probed with HIV-specific antigens. Positive results are indicated by distinct bands corresponding to specific HIV antigens.
- **Clinical Utility**: Western blot is considered the gold standard confirmatory test for HIV diagnosis, providing definitive evidence of HIV infection following reactive screening results. Interpretation involves strict criteria for band intensity and specificity to minimize indeterminate results and

ensure accurate diagnosis.

2. Immunofluorescence Assay (IFA)

- **Principle**: Immunofluorescence assay detects HIV-specific antibodies (IgM/IgG) in serum or plasma samples using fluorescent-labeled antigens (e.g., gp160, gp120, p24) for visual detection under fluorescence microscopy.
- **Procedure**: Serum or plasma samples are incubated with fluorescent-labeled HIV antigens, followed by microscopic examination for specific antibody-antigen interactions. Positive results are visualized as fluorescent patterns indicative of HIV-specific antibody binding.
- **Clinical Utility**: IFA serves as an alternative confirmatory test to Western blot, providing qualitative detection of HIV-specific antibodies with high sensitivity and specificity. Results complement initial screening assays and guide clinical decisions regarding HIV diagnosis and management.

3. Line Immunoassay (LIA)

- **Principle**: Line immunoassay detects HIV-specific antibodies (IgM/IgG) against multiple viral antigens (e.g., gp160, gp120, p24) in serum or plasma samples using antigen-coated strips for antibody binding and visualization.
- **Procedure**: Serum or plasma samples are incubated with antigen-coated strips, allowing specific antibody-antigen interactions. Positive results are indicated by visible lines corresponding to specific HIV antigens, facilitating qualitative confirmation of HIV infection.
- **Clinical Utility**: LIA combines the advantages of Western blot and immunofluorescence assays, offering rapid, reliable, and user-friendly confirmatory testing for HIV diagnosis in diverse healthcare settings.

Interpretation guidelines ensure accurate diagnosis and differentiation of true HIV infection from cross-reactive antibody responses.

Viral Load Measurement in HIV Management

Viral load measurement quantifies the concentration of HIV RNA in blood plasma, providing critical insights into viral replication dynamics, treatment response, and disease progression monitoring:

Principle and Methodology

- **Quantitative PCR (qPCR)**: Viral load testing utilizes quantitative PCR to amplify and quantify HIV RNA in blood plasma samples, providing accurate measurement of viral replication levels over time.
- **Clinical Indications**: Viral load measurement informs clinical decision-making in HIV management, including ART initiation, treatment response assessment, and detection of virological failure (e.g., persistent viral replication despite adherence to ART).
- **Thresholds and Interpretation**: Viral load thresholds (e.g., <50 copies/mL) guide therapeutic goals for achieving viral suppression, reducing the risk of disease progression, and preventing HIV transmission to uninfected partners.

Clinical Implications of Confirmatory Tests and Viral Load Measurement

Confirmatory tests and viral load measurement contribute to comprehensive HIV/AIDS care, influencing diagnostic accuracy, treatment decisions, and patient outcomes:

- **Diagnosis Confirmation**: Confirmatory tests (e.g., Western blot, LIA) verify HIV infection following initial screening, ensuring accurate diagnosis and facilitating timely initiation of ART to optimize clinical outcomes.
- **Treatment Initiation**: Viral load measurement guides

ART initiation based on virological thresholds, promoting early viral suppression, preserving immune function, and reducing the risk of AIDS-related complications.

- **Monitoring Disease Progression**: Regular viral load monitoring assesses treatment efficacy, detects virological rebound, and informs therapeutic adjustments to achieve sustained viral suppression and long-term HIV/AIDS management.
- **Prevention of HIV Transmission**: Viral load suppression through effective ART reduces HIV transmission risk to uninfected partners, supporting HIV prevention strategies (e.g., Treatment as Prevention) and contributing to epidemic control efforts.

Innovations and Future Directions

Advancements in HIV diagnostics and viral load monitoring continue to shape clinical practice and public health strategies:

- **Point-of-Care Testing**: Integration of POC assays for confirmatory testing and viral load measurement enhances accessibility, facilitates decentralized HIV testing services, and promotes early diagnosis and treatment initiation in underserved communities.
- **Next-Generation Assays**: Development of novel diagnostic platforms (e.g., digital immunoassays, multiplex serological assays) improves assay sensitivity, specificity, and throughput for enhanced HIV screening and monitoring capabilities.
- **Implementation Science**: Implementation science research evaluates the impact of diagnostic innovations, screening algorithms, and viral load monitoring strategies on HIV/AIDS care outcomes, informing evidence-based practices and healthcare policy development.

Conclusion

Confirmatory tests and viral load measurement are integral components of HIV diagnosis, treatment, and monitoring strategies, providing essential clinical insights into disease progression, treatment response, and virological control. Understanding the principles, methodologies, clinical implications, and advancements in confirmatory testing and viral load measurement is crucial for healthcare providers, policymakers, and stakeholders involved in HIV/AIDS prevention, care, and management. Comprehensive approaches integrating innovative diagnostics, public health interventions, and community engagement efforts are essential in achieving universal access to accurate HIV diagnosis, optimizing treatment outcomes, and advancing towards global HIV/AIDS epidemic control and elimination goals.

CD4 Count and Immunological Monitoring in HIV/AIDS

CD4 count and immunological monitoring play crucial roles in assessing immune function, guiding clinical management decisions, and monitoring disease progression in individuals living with Human Immunodeficiency Virus (HIV) infection and Acquired Immunodeficiency Syndrome (AIDS). This section explores the principles, methodologies, clinical implications, and advancements in CD4 count measurement and immunological monitoring, highlighting their significance in HIV/AIDS care.

Introduction to CD4 Count and Immunological Monitoring

CD4 T-cells are essential components of the immune system involved in orchestrating immune responses against pathogens, including HIV. CD4 count measurement serves as a surrogate marker for immune function, guiding therapeutic decisions and predicting the risk of opportunistic infections and AIDS-related complications in HIV-infected individuals.

Principles of CD4 Count Measurement

CD4 count measurement involves quantifying the number of CD4-positive T-cells per microliter (μL) of blood, providing insights into immune status and disease progression in HIV/AIDS:

- **Flow Cytometry**: Flow cytometry is the gold standard method for CD4 count measurement, utilizing fluorescently labeled antibodies against CD4 antigens to enumerate CD4 T-cells in whole blood or peripheral blood mononuclear cells (PBMCs).

- **Clinical Relevance**: CD4 count reflects immune function and helps stratify HIV-infected individuals into different clinical stages (e.g., acute infection, chronic infection, AIDS), guiding treatment initiation, prophylactic interventions, and monitoring of disease progression over time.

- **Thresholds and Interpretation**: CD4 count thresholds (e.g., <200 cells/μL) define immunological categories (e.g., immunocompetent, immunodeficient) and inform clinical decisions regarding opportunistic infection prophylaxis, vaccination strategies, and ART initiation.

Immunological Monitoring in HIV/AIDS

Immunological monitoring encompasses comprehensive assessments of immune function, including CD4 count measurement, immune activation markers, and cytokine profiles, to optimize HIV/AIDS management strategies:

- **Biomarkers of Immune Activation**: Monitoring immune activation markers (e.g., CD38, HLA-DR expression on T-cells) and inflammatory cytokines (e.g., IL-6, TNF-alpha) provides insights into HIV-associated immune dysregulation, chronic inflammation, and cardiovascular comorbidities.

- **Immune Reconstitution**: ART-mediated immune

reconstitution involves restoration of CD4 T-cell counts, normalization of immune activation markers, and preservation of immune responses against opportunistic pathogens, improving clinical outcomes and quality of life.

Clinical Implications of CD4 Count and Immunological Monitoring

CD4 count measurement and immunological monitoring inform clinical decision-making, therapeutic strategies, and long-term management of HIV/AIDS:

- **ART Initiation**: CD4 count-guided ART initiation (e.g., <350 cells/µL based on WHO guidelines) prevents immune deterioration, reduces HIV replication, and enhances immune recovery to achieve sustained viral suppression and improve clinical outcomes.
- **Opportunistic Infection Prophylaxis**: CD4-guided prophylactic interventions (e.g., trimethoprim-sulfamethoxazole for PCP prophylaxis) reduce the risk of opportunistic infections and AIDS-related morbidity/mortality in immunocompromised individuals.
- **Disease Monitoring**: Serial CD4 count monitoring assesses ART efficacy, predicts the risk of AIDS-related complications (e.g., opportunistic infections, AIDS-defining cancers), and guides therapeutic adjustments to optimize treatment outcomes and prevent disease progression.

Advancements in CD4 Count Technology

Advancements in CD4 count technology aim to enhance assay sensitivity, accuracy, and accessibility in diverse healthcare settings:

- **Point-of-Care Testing (POC)**: POC CD4 assays facilitate decentralized testing, rapid result turnaround, and immediate clinical decision-making in resource-limited settings, improving access to CD4 monitoring and HIV/AIDS care services.

- **Flow Cytometry Innovations**: Automated flow cytometry platforms integrate multiparametric analysis, high throughput, and enhanced sensitivity for precise CD4 count quantification, supporting large-scale immunological monitoring programs and research initiatives.

Integration of CD4 Monitoring in HIV/AIDS Care

Integration of CD4 monitoring in comprehensive HIV/AIDS care involves multidisciplinary approaches, including:

- **Treatment Adherence**: Regular CD4 monitoring encourages treatment adherence, supports patient engagement in HIV care, and fosters collaboration between healthcare providers and individuals living with HIV/AIDS.
- **Clinical Decision Support**: CD4-based clinical algorithms guide therapeutic decisions (e.g., ART initiation, opportunistic infection management) tailored to individual immune status, treatment response, and comorbidities.

Future Directions in Immunological Monitoring

Future directions in immunological monitoring focus on personalized medicine approaches, immune-based interventions, and innovative technologies to optimize HIV/AIDS management and achieve sustained viral suppression:

- **Precision Medicine**: Integration of biomarkers (e.g., CD4 count, immune activation markers) and genomic profiling informs personalized treatment strategies, identifies host factors influencing HIV pathogenesis, and enhances therapeutic outcomes in HIV-infected individuals.
- **Immune-Based Therapies**: Development of immune-modulatory therapies (e.g., therapeutic vaccines,

immune checkpoint inhibitors) targets HIV reservoirs, enhances immune responses, and achieves functional cure or long-term viral remission in selected patient populations.

Conclusion

CD4 count measurement and immunological monitoring are essential components of HIV/AIDS care, providing critical insights into immune status, disease progression, and therapeutic efficacy. Understanding the principles, methodologies, clinical implications, and advancements in CD4 monitoring and immunological assessments is fundamental for healthcare providers, researchers, and policymakers involved in HIV/AIDS prevention, treatment, and management. Comprehensive strategies integrating CD4 monitoring with ART initiation, opportunistic infection prophylaxis, and personalized healthcare approaches contribute to improved clinical outcomes, enhanced quality of life, and progress towards global HIV/AIDS epidemic control and elimination goals.

CHAPTER 6: TREATMENT AND MANAGEMENT

Antiretroviral Therapy (ART)

Antiretroviral therapy (ART) revolutionized the management of Human Immunodeficiency Virus (HIV) infection, transforming it from a fatal disease to a chronic manageable condition. This section explores the principles, classes of antiretroviral drugs, initiation and adherence strategies, and management of treatment failure in ART for HIV/AIDS.

Introduction to Antiretroviral Therapy (ART)

Antiretroviral therapy (ART) refers to the use of combinations of antiretroviral drugs to suppress HIV replication, preserve immune function, and prevent disease progression in individuals living with HIV/AIDS. The goals of ART include achieving sustained viral suppression, restoring immune competence, reducing HIV-associated morbidity and mortality, and preventing HIV transmission to uninfected individuals.

Historical Perspective and Evolution of ART

The development of ART marked a pivotal milestone in the history of HIV/AIDS treatment, characterized by:

- **Discovery of HIV**: Identification of HIV as the causative agent of AIDS in the early 1980s led to intensive research efforts to develop effective antiretroviral therapies targeting different stages of the HIV life cycle.

- **Introduction of Mono and Dual Therapy**: Initial treatment strategies involved monotherapy with nucleoside reverse transcriptase inhibitors (NRTIs) such as zidovudine (AZT). Dual therapy combinations (e.g., AZT + lamivudine) followed, demonstrating improved virological control but limited durability due to viral resistance.
- **Advances in Combination Therapy**: The advent of combination antiretroviral therapy (cART) in the mid-1990s, combining drugs from different classes, revolutionized HIV treatment by significantly reducing viral load, restoring immune function, and prolonging survival.
- **Lifelong Treatment Paradigm**: ART is currently recommended as lifelong therapy, requiring adherence to suppress viral replication, prevent drug resistance, and maintain long-term health outcomes for individuals living with HIV/AIDS.

Classes of Antiretroviral Drugs

Antiretroviral drugs target distinct stages of the HIV life cycle, inhibiting viral replication and reducing viral load to undetectable levels. The classes of antiretroviral drugs include:

1. Nucleoside/Nucleotide Reverse Transcriptase Inhibitors (NRTIs/NtRTIs)

- **Mechanism of Action**: NRTIs/NtRTIs inhibit HIV reverse transcriptase enzyme, blocking viral RNA to DNA conversion and halting viral replication.
- **Examples**: Zidovudine (AZT), lamivudine (3TC), tenofovir disoproxil fumarate (TDF), tenofovir alafenamide (TAF), abacavir (ABC).
- **Clinical Use**: Backbone of most cART regimens due to efficacy, safety profile, and low pill burden. TAF is preferred over TDF due to renal and bone safety.

2. Non-Nucleoside Reverse Transcriptase Inhibitors (NNRTIs)

- **Mechanism of Action**: NNRTIs bind directly to HIV reverse transcriptase, preventing RNA to DNA conversion and viral replication.
- **Examples**: Efavirenz (EFV), nevirapine (NVP), rilpivirine (RPV).
- **Clinical Use**: Oral administration, convenient dosing, and potency against HIV-1 strains. EFV is less favored due to central nervous system side effects.

3. Protease Inhibitors (PIs)

- **Mechanism of Action**: PIs block HIV protease enzyme, preventing cleavage of viral polyprotein precursors and inhibiting viral maturation.
- **Examples**: Lopinavir/ritonavir (LPV/r), atazanavir (ATV), darunavir (DRV).
- **Clinical Use**: Used in combination with NRTIs as potent second-line or salvage therapy. Boosted PIs (e.g., LPV/r) enhance pharmacokinetics and efficacy.

4. Integrase Strand Transfer Inhibitors (INSTIs)

- **Mechanism of Action**: INSTIs inhibit integrase enzyme, preventing integration of viral DNA into host cell genome and halting viral replication.
- **Examples**: Raltegravir (RAL), dolutegravir (DTG), bictegravir (BIC).
- **Clinical Use**: Preferred first-line therapy due to high potency, rapid viral suppression, and favorable tolerability. DTG is recommended in treatment-naive and treatment-experienced patients.

5. Entry Inhibitors

- **Mechanism of Action**: Entry inhibitors block viral entry into host cells by targeting HIV envelope glycoproteins (gp41 or CCR5 coreceptor).
- **Examples**: Maraviroc (CCR5 antagonist), enfuvirtide

(fusion inhibitor).
- **Clinical Use**: Reserved for salvage therapy in individuals with multidrug-resistant HIV or viral tropism testing showing CCR5-tropic virus.

6. **Pharmacokinetic Enhancers**
   - **Mechanism of Action**: Pharmacokinetic enhancers (e.g., ritonavir, cobicistat) boost plasma concentrations of other antiretroviral drugs by inhibiting drug-metabolizing enzymes (e.g., CYP3A4).
   - **Clinical Use**: Enhance bioavailability and half-life of PIs and INSTIs in cART regimens, reducing pill burden and dosing frequency.

Combination Antiretroviral Therapy (cART)

Effective ART involves combining drugs from different classes (cART), targeting multiple stages of the HIV life cycle to achieve sustained viral suppression, prevent drug resistance, and preserve immune function. Principles of cART include:
- **Regimen Selection**: Tailoring cART regimens based on individual factors (e.g., baseline viral load, drug resistance testing, comorbidities) to optimize efficacy, tolerability, and adherence.
- **Fixed-Dose Combinations (FDCs)**: FDCs combine multiple antiretroviral drugs into single-pill formulations, simplifying dosing, improving adherence, and reducing pill burden for patients on lifelong therapy.
- **Adherence Strategies**: Promoting adherence through patient education, counseling, adherence support programs, and innovative drug delivery systems (e.g., long-acting formulations, POC devices) to optimize treatment outcomes and prevent virological failure.

Initiation and Adherence to ART

Initiation and adherence to ART are critical determinants of treatment success, viral suppression, and long-term health outcomes in HIV-infected individuals:

Initiation of ART

- **Clinical Guidelines**: Initiation of ART is guided by clinical guidelines (e.g., WHO, DHHS) recommending early treatment initiation regardless of CD4 count (e.g., <350 cells/µL) to prevent disease progression, reduce transmission risk, and improve survival.
- **Baseline Evaluation**: Baseline evaluation includes comprehensive assessment of HIV disease stage, viral load, CD4 count, HIV drug resistance testing, hepatitis B/C coinfection status, and assessment of comorbidities to inform personalized treatment decisions.
- **Treatment Regimen Selection**: Selection of initial ART regimen considers drug efficacy, safety profile, drug-drug interactions, patient preferences, and adherence potential. Preferred regimens often include INSTIs or integrase-based combinations due to high potency, rapid viral suppression, and favorable tolerability.

Adherence to ART

- **Barriers to Adherence**: Barriers to adherence include pill burden, adverse effects, comorbidities, substance use, mental health issues, stigma, socioeconomic factors, and healthcare access.
- **Adherence Strategies**: Multifaceted adherence strategies include patient education, counseling, medication reminders, pill organizers, digital health technologies (e.g., smartphone apps), peer support groups, and community-based interventions to enhance medication adherence and retention in HIV care.
- **Monitoring and Support**: Regular monitoring of viral load, CD4 count, and medication adherence

assessments informs clinical decision-making, identifies adherence challenges, and facilitates timely interventions (e.g., adherence counseling, regimen simplification) to optimize treatment outcomes.

Management of Treatment Failure

Management of treatment failure involves comprehensive evaluation, identification of contributing factors, and adjustment of ART regimens to achieve viral suppression and preserve immune function:

Virological Failure

- **Definition**: Virological failure is defined as persistent HIV RNA >200 copies/mL after at least 6 months of ART, indicating inadequate viral suppression and potential development of drug resistance mutations.
- **Causes**: Causes of virological failure include poor medication adherence, drug interactions, suboptimal ART potency, viral resistance mutations, pharmacokinetic variability, and comorbidities affecting drug absorption or metabolism.
- **Diagnostic Evaluation**: Diagnostic evaluation includes repeat viral load testing, drug resistance testing (genotypic/phenotypic), adherence assessments, clinical evaluation for opportunistic infections, and assessment of drug-drug interactions.

Management Strategies

- **Regimen Optimization**: Regimen optimization involves switching to a new ART regimen based on drug resistance testing, treatment history, and individualized factors (e.g., comorbidities, tolerability) to enhance virological suppression and prevent further resistance.
- **Enhanced Adherence Support**: Intensified adherence support interventions (e.g., adherence counseling, medication adherence aids, treatment literacy)

address adherence barriers, promote medication adherence, and improve treatment outcomes in individuals experiencing virological failure.
- **Second-line and Salvage Therapy**: Second-line ART regimens include alternative drug classes (e.g., boosted PIs, second-generation INSTIs) with activity against resistant HIV strains, aiming to achieve durable viral suppression and preserve treatment options for future therapy.

Multidisciplinary Care Approach
- **Collaborative Care**: Multidisciplinary care teams (e.g., infectious disease specialists, pharmacists, nurses, social workers) collaborate to optimize treatment adherence, monitor treatment response, manage comorbidities, and support psychosocial well-being in patients with treatment failure.

Advancements in ART and Future Directions

Advancements in ART focus on improving treatment outcomes, reducing treatment complexity, enhancing drug tolerability, and expanding therapeutic options:
- **Long-acting Formulations**: Development of long-acting injectable formulations (e.g., cabotegravir, rilpivirine) provides extended dosing intervals (e.g., monthly) for improved convenience, adherence, and treatment adherence in select patient populations.
- **Novel Drug Targets**: Exploration of novel drug targets (e.g., HIV entry inhibitors, maturation inhibitors, broadly neutralizing antibodies) targets persistent viral reservoirs, enhances immune responses, and explores potential strategies for HIV cure research.
- **Personalized Medicine Approaches**: Integration of biomarkers (e.g., drug resistance testing, pharmacogenomics) and precision medicine approaches tailor ART regimens to individual patient

characteristics, optimizing treatment efficacy, safety, and long-term adherence.

Conclusion

Antiretroviral therapy (ART) represents a cornerstone in the management of HIV/AIDS, transforming a once fatal disease into a chronic manageable condition characterized by sustained viral suppression, immune restoration, and improved quality of life. Understanding the principles, classes of antiretroviral drugs, initiation strategies, adherence challenges, and management of treatment failure is essential for healthcare providers, researchers, and policymakers involved in HIV/AIDS care. Comprehensive approaches integrating ART with adherence support, viral monitoring, and multidisciplinary care facilitate optimal treatment outcomes, mitigate virological failure, and advance global efforts towards achieving universal access to effective HIV/AIDS treatment, care, and prevention strategies.

Opportunistic Infection Prophylaxis and Treatment in HIV/AIDS

Opportunistic infections (OIs) remain a significant cause of morbidity and mortality in individuals living with Human Immunodeficiency Virus (HIV) infection, particularly those with advanced immunosuppression. Effective prophylaxis and treatment of OIs are essential components of comprehensive HIV/AIDS care to reduce disease burden, prevent complications, and improve clinical outcomes. This section explores the principles, strategies, and specific interventions for opportunistic infection prophylaxis and treatment in HIV/AIDS.

Introduction to Opportunistic Infections in HIV/AIDS

Opportunistic infections are caused by pathogens that typically do not cause disease in immunocompetent individuals but exploit weakened immune defenses in HIV-infected individuals with reduced CD4 T-cell counts. Common opportunistic infections include bacterial, fungal, viral, and parasitic pathogens, presenting with diverse clinical manifestations and varying degrees of severity depending on the degree of immunosuppression.

Principles of Opportunistic Infection Prophylaxis

Opportunistic infection prophylaxis aims to prevent initial infection or reactivation of latent infections in HIV-infected individuals, particularly those with CD4 T-cell counts below specific thresholds:

- **CD4 Thresholds**: Prophylaxis guidelines are based on CD4 T-cell counts and include initiation, duration, and discontinuation criteria to optimize efficacy and minimize risks of drug toxicity and resistance.
- **Individualized Approach**: Prophylactic strategies are tailored based on individual risk factors (e.g., geographic location, immunization status, prior OI history, ART regimen) to prioritize interventions and optimize clinical outcomes.

Common Opportunistic Infections and Prophylactic Strategies

1. Pneumocystis jirovecii Pneumonia (PCP)

- **Prophylaxis**: Trimethoprim-sulfamethoxazole (TMP-SMX) is the preferred agent for primary and secondary PCP prophylaxis in HIV-infected individuals with CD4 counts <200 cells/µL or a history of oropharyngeal candidiasis.
- **Alternative Agents**: Alternative regimens include dapsone, atovaquone, or aerosolized pentamidine based on patient tolerance, allergies, or contraindications to TMP-SMX.

2. Mycobacterium avium Complex (MAC)

- **Prophylaxis**: Azithromycin or clarithromycin is recommended for MAC prophylaxis in individuals with CD4 counts <50 cells/µL to prevent disseminated disease.

3. Tuberculosis (TB)

- **Prophylaxis**: Isoniazid (INH) prophylaxis is indicated in HIV-infected individuals with latent TB infection (LTBI) and no evidence of active TB disease, irrespective of CD4 count, to reduce the risk of TB reactivation.

4. Cryptococcal Meningitis

- **Prophylaxis**: Fluconazole is recommended for primary prophylaxis against cryptococcal infection in HIV-infected individuals with CD4 counts <100 cells/µL.

5. Toxoplasmosis

- **Prophylaxis**: Trimethoprim-sulfamethoxazole (TMP-SMX) is recommended for primary prophylaxis against toxoplasmosis in HIV-infected individuals with CD4 counts <100 cells/µL and positive toxoplasma serology.

Treatment of Opportunistic Infections

Prompt diagnosis and effective treatment of OIs are critical to reduce morbidity, mortality, and disease progression in HIV-infected individuals:

1. Antibacterial Therapy

- **Common Infections**: Treatment of bacterial infections (e.g., bacterial pneumonia, bacterial enteritis) involves empirical antibiotic therapy targeting common pathogens, adjusting based on culture and susceptibility results.

2. Antifungal Therapy

- **Cryptococcal Meningitis**: Induction therapy with amphotericin B plus flucytosine followed by consolidation and maintenance therapy with fluconazole for cryptococcal meningitis.
- **Candidiasis**: Fluconazole or alternative azoles are

used for the treatment of esophageal candidiasis or oropharyngeal candidiasis.

3. Antiviral Therapy

- **Herpes Simplex Virus (HSV)**: Acyclovir, valacyclovir, or famciclovir are used for treatment and suppression of HSV infections.
- **Cytomegalovirus (CMV)**: Ganciclovir or valganciclovir are used for the treatment of CMV retinitis or other CMV manifestations.

4. Antiparasitic Therapy

- **Toxoplasmosis**: Treatment with pyrimethamine plus sulfadiazine and leucovorin for toxoplasmic encephalitis.
- **Cryptosporidiosis**: Supportive therapy along with nitazoxanide or paromomycin for cryptosporidiosis.

Management Strategies for Opportunistic Infection Prophylaxis and Treatment

1. Multidisciplinary Approach

- **Collaborative Care**: Multidisciplinary teams (e.g., infectious disease specialists, pharmacists, nurses) collaborate to optimize prophylactic interventions, ensure timely diagnosis, and implement evidence-based treatment strategies for OIs.

2. Integrated Care

- **Integration with ART**: Opportunistic infection prophylaxis and treatment are integrated with ART initiation and adherence support to achieve comprehensive HIV/AIDS management, reduce disease complications, and improve long-term clinical outcomes.

3. Monitoring and Surveillance

- **Virological and Immunological Monitoring**: Regular monitoring of CD4 counts, viral load, and immune function informs clinical decision-making, assesses treatment response, and identifies individuals at risk for OIs requiring prophylaxis or treatment.

4. Health Education and Prevention

- **Patient Education**: Health education initiatives promote awareness of opportunistic infections, adherence to prophylactic regimens, early recognition of symptoms, and timely healthcare-seeking behaviors among HIV-infected individuals.

Advances and Future Directions

Advancements in HIV/AIDS care focus on optimizing prophylactic strategies, expanding treatment options, and integrating novel therapies to improve outcomes and quality of life:

- **Long-acting Prophylactic Therapies**: Development of long-acting formulations (e.g., injectable antifungals, antivirals) for prophylaxis against OIs offers convenience, adherence support, and potential for reducing treatment burden in HIV-infected populations.
- **Precision Medicine Approaches**: Integration of biomarkers (e.g., CD4 counts, viral load, immune activation markers) and genomic profiling informs personalized prophylactic strategies, enhances treatment efficacy, and identifies individuals at high risk for OIs.
- **Global Health Initiatives**: Scaling up access to prophylactic interventions, diagnostic technologies, and effective treatments for OIs in resource-limited settings strengthens healthcare infrastructure, reduces disparities, and supports global efforts towards HIV/AIDS epidemic control and elimination.

Conclusion

Opportunistic infection prophylaxis and treatment are essential components of comprehensive HIV/AIDS care, aiming to reduce disease burden, prevent complications, and improve clinical outcomes in immunocompromised individuals. Understanding the principles, strategies, and specific interventions for OI prophylaxis and treatment is crucial for healthcare providers, researchers, and policymakers involved in HIV/AIDS management. Integrated approaches combining ART with targeted prophylactic regimens, adherence support, multidisciplinary care, and innovative therapeutic strategies contribute to achieving sustained viral suppression, enhancing immune function, and advancing towards universal access to effective HIV/AIDS treatment and care worldwide.

Immunomodulatory Therapies in HIV/AIDS

Immunomodulatory therapies play a crucial role in the management of Human Immunodeficiency Virus (HIV) infection by enhancing immune responses, reducing chronic inflammation, and potentially influencing disease progression and outcomes. This section explores the principles, mechanisms of action, clinical applications, and future perspectives of immunomodulatory therapies in HIV/AIDS.

Introduction to Immunomodulatory Therapies

Immunomodulatory therapies encompass a diverse range of interventions designed to modify or regulate immune responses in individuals living with HIV/AIDS. These therapies aim to restore immune function, mitigate immune dysregulation, and optimize immune responses against HIV and opportunistic infections.

Mechanisms of Action

Immunomodulatory therapies exert their effects through various mechanisms, including:

- **Immune Activation**: Stimulating immune responses to enhance antiviral immunity and immune surveillance against HIV-infected cells.

- **Immune Suppression**: Suppressing hyperactive immune responses or chronic inflammation to mitigate immune-mediated tissue damage and improve overall immune function.
- **Anti-inflammatory Effects**: Modulating cytokine profiles and reducing systemic inflammation associated with HIV infection and immune activation.

Types of Immunomodulatory Therapies

1. Interleukin Therapies

- **Interleukin-2 (IL-2)**: IL-2 therapy aims to expand CD4 and CD8 T-cell populations, enhance immune function, and potentially delay disease progression in HIV-infected individuals with suboptimal immune recovery despite antiretroviral therapy (ART).
- **Clinical Applications**: IL-2 therapy is investigated in clinical trials to evaluate its efficacy in combination with ART in improving immune reconstitution and reducing HIV reservoirs.

2. Cytokine Modulators

- **Tumor Necrosis Factor (TNF) Inhibitors**: TNF inhibitors (e.g., etanercept) are investigated for their potential to reduce chronic inflammation and immune activation in HIV-infected individuals, although safety concerns and risk of opportunistic infections limit their widespread use.
- **Interferons**: Interferon-alpha (IFN-α) has antiviral properties and modulates immune responses, explored in HIV cure research to activate latent HIV reservoirs and enhance immune surveillance against persistent infection.

3. Thymic Growth Factors

- **Thymopentin**: Thymopentin stimulates thymic

function and T-cell production, potentially enhancing immune reconstitution in HIV-infected individuals with impaired thymic output due to chronic HIV infection or aging.
- **Clinical Applications**: Thymopentin is investigated in clinical studies to assess its role in improving CD4 T-cell recovery and immune function in combination with ART.

4. Anti-inflammatory Agents
- **Corticosteroids**: Corticosteroids are used in the management of immune-mediated complications (e.g., immune reconstitution inflammatory syndrome [IRIS]) in HIV-infected individuals initiating ART, reducing inflammation and tissue damage associated with immune recovery.
- **Clinical Applications**: Short-term use of corticosteroids may mitigate severe IRIS manifestations, although prolonged use is limited by adverse effects and potential for opportunistic infections.

Clinical Applications and Considerations

1. Enhancement of Immune Reconstitution
- Immunomodulatory therapies aim to augment CD4 T-cell recovery and immune reconstitution in individuals with suboptimal responses to ART, potentially reducing risks of opportunistic infections and non-AIDS-related complications.

2. Management of Immune Activation and Inflammation
- Targeting chronic immune activation and inflammation in HIV infection may mitigate risks of cardiovascular disease, neurocognitive impairment, and other inflammatory-driven comorbidities associated with persistent viral replication and immune dysregulation.

3. Integration with Antiretroviral Therapy (ART)
- Immunomodulatory therapies are integrated with ART to optimize treatment outcomes, enhance immune responses, and reduce HIV reservoirs, supporting comprehensive HIV/AIDS management strategies.

Future Perspectives and Research Directions

Advancements in immunomodulatory therapies focus on personalized medicine approaches, novel targets, and combination therapies to improve efficacy, safety, and long-term outcomes in HIV/AIDS:

- **Precision Medicine**: Integration of biomarkers (e.g., immune activation markers, viral reservoirs) and genomic profiling informs personalized immunomodulatory strategies tailored to individual immune profiles and treatment responses.
- **Novel Therapeutic Targets**: Exploration of novel immune checkpoints, cytokine signaling pathways, and immunoregulatory mechanisms offers potential targets for developing next-generation immunomodulatory therapies in HIV/AIDS.
- **Clinical Trials and Innovation**: Continued clinical trials and translational research initiatives evaluate the safety, efficacy, and therapeutic benefits of immunomodulatory interventions in diverse HIV-infected populations, addressing unmet medical needs and advancing towards HIV cure research.

Conclusion

Immunomodulatory therapies represent promising adjunctive approaches in the management of HIV/AIDS, aiming to restore immune function, mitigate immune dysregulation, and optimize treatment outcomes in individuals living with HIV infection. Understanding the mechanisms, clinical applications, and future directions of immunomodulatory therapies is crucial for healthcare providers, researchers, and policymakers involved in HIV/AIDS care, supporting integrated strategies to achieve sustained viral suppression, immune reconstitution, and improved quality of life for individuals affected by HIV/AIDS globally.

Supportive Care and Holistic Approaches in HIV/AIDS

Supportive care and holistic approaches are integral components of comprehensive HIV/AIDS management, aiming to optimize quality of life, address multifaceted needs, and enhance overall well-being for individuals living with Human Immunodeficiency Virus (HIV) infection. This section explores the principles, strategies, and specific interventions encompassing nutritional support, mental health services, and counseling within the context of HIV/AIDS care.

Introduction to Supportive Care in HIV/AIDS

Supportive care encompasses a broad spectrum of interventions designed to address physical, psychological, social, and spiritual needs of individuals affected by HIV/AIDS. These interventions complement medical treatments such as antiretroviral therapy (ART), aiming to improve treatment adherence, mitigate complications, and promote holistic well-being across the continuum of HIV care.

Principles of Supportive Care

Supportive care in HIV/AIDS is guided by principles that emphasize:

- **Comprehensive Assessment**: Holistic assessment of individual needs, including physical health, psychosocial well-being, socioeconomic factors, and cultural considerations, to tailor personalized supportive care interventions.
- **Multidisciplinary Collaboration**: Collaborative care involving healthcare providers (e.g., physicians,

nurses, psychologists, social workers), community organizations, and support networks to address diverse patient needs and optimize treatment outcomes.
- **Patient-Centered Approach**: Empowering patients as active participants in their care, fostering open communication, shared decision-making, and respect for individual preferences, values, and goals.

Nutritional Support

Nutritional support plays a crucial role in HIV/AIDS care, influencing immune function, treatment outcomes, and overall quality of life for individuals living with HIV infection. Effective nutritional interventions aim to address nutritional deficiencies, promote optimal health outcomes, and mitigate complications associated with HIV/AIDS and its treatment.

Nutritional Needs in HIV/AIDS

- **Energy Requirements**: Individuals with HIV/AIDS may have increased energy requirements due to metabolic demands, chronic inflammation, and opportunistic infections, necessitating adequate caloric intake to support immune function and disease management.
- **Micronutrient Deficiencies**: HIV infection is associated with micronutrient deficiencies (e.g., vitamin D, vitamin B12, zinc), contributing to immune dysfunction, oxidative stress, and disease progression.
- **Protein and Amino Acids**: Protein malnutrition or deficiency can impair immune responses, muscle mass, and functional status in HIV-infected individuals, highlighting the importance of adequate protein intake for overall health and well-being.

Strategies for Nutritional Support

- **Dietary Counseling**: Individualized dietary counseling by registered dietitians or nutritionists promotes balanced nutrition, encourages adherence to

recommended dietary guidelines, and addresses specific nutritional needs based on HIV disease stage, comorbidities, and ART regimen.
- **Micronutrient Supplementation**: Supplementation with essential micronutrients (e.g., multivitamins, vitamin D, zinc) may be recommended to correct deficiencies, support immune function, and improve treatment outcomes in HIV/AIDS.
- **Enteral and Parenteral Nutrition**: Enteral nutrition via oral nutritional supplements or tube feeding and parenteral nutrition may be considered for individuals with severe malnutrition, swallowing difficulties, or gastrointestinal complications impairing nutrient absorption.
- **Food Security and Access**: Addressing food insecurity through social support programs, food assistance initiatives, and community resources enhances nutritional outcomes and promotes treatment adherence among socioeconomically vulnerable populations affected by HIV/AIDS.

Impact of Nutritional Support on HIV/AIDS Outcomes
- **Immune Function**: Optimal nutrition supports immune reconstitution, enhances CD4 T-cell recovery, and reduces susceptibility to opportunistic infections in HIV-infected individuals receiving ART.
- **Treatment Adherence**: Improved nutritional status correlates with enhanced treatment adherence, reduced medication side effects, and improved tolerability of ART regimens, contributing to sustained viral suppression and long-term clinical stability.
- **Quality of Life**: Comprehensive nutritional support improves overall quality of life, physical functioning, and nutritional well-being in individuals living with HIV/AIDS, promoting independence, self-

management, and psychosocial resilience.

Mental Health and Counseling

Mental health and psychosocial support are critical components of HIV/AIDS care, addressing the emotional, psychological, and social challenges experienced by individuals affected by HIV infection. Integrated mental health services and counseling interventions aim to enhance coping mechanisms, improve treatment adherence, and promote holistic well-being across the lifespan.

Mental Health Challenges in HIV/AIDS

- **Psychological Distress**: Diagnosis of HIV/AIDS may evoke feelings of fear, anxiety, depression, grief, and stigma, impacting mental health, treatment engagement, and quality of life.
- **Neurocognitive Disorders**: HIV-associated neurocognitive disorders (HAND) encompass a spectrum of cognitive impairments, ranging from mild neurocognitive deficits to severe dementia, affecting functional independence and daily living activities.
- **Substance Use Disorders**: Co-occurring substance use disorders (e.g., alcohol, illicit drugs) are prevalent among individuals with HIV/AIDS, exacerbating treatment adherence challenges, disease progression, and comorbid health conditions.

Strategies for Mental Health and Counseling

- **Psychosocial Assessment**: Comprehensive psychosocial assessment evaluates mental health status, identifies psychosocial stressors, assesses coping resources, and informs individualized treatment planning in HIV/AIDS care.
- **Cognitive Behavioral Therapy (CBT)**: CBT interventions target maladaptive thoughts, behaviors, and emotional responses associated with HIV/AIDS-

related stress, depression, and anxiety, promoting adaptive coping strategies and resilience.

- **Supportive Counseling**: Individual or group counseling provides a safe space for emotional expression, validation of experiences, psychoeducation on HIV/AIDS, and skill-building in stress management, communication, and decision-making.
- **Peer Support Programs**: Peer-led support groups and community-based networks offer peer support, mutual encouragement, and shared experiences among individuals affected by HIV/AIDS, fostering social connectedness and reducing isolation.

Integrated Care Models

- **Collaborative Care**: Integrated models of care involving collaboration between mental health professionals, HIV specialists, primary care providers, and community organizations optimize treatment outcomes, address comorbidities, and promote continuity of care.
- **Trauma-Informed Care**: Trauma-informed approaches recognize and respond to the impact of past trauma on mental health, substance use, and overall well-being, promoting healing, empowerment, and recovery in individuals living with HIV/AIDS.

Impact of Mental Health and Counseling on HIV/AIDS Outcomes

- **Treatment Adherence**: Effective mental health support and counseling improve treatment adherence, medication management, and retention in HIV care, reducing risks of virological failure and emergence of drug resistance.
- **Quality of Life**: Psychosocial interventions enhance quality of life, emotional resilience, and psychosocial

well-being in individuals affected by HIV/AIDS, promoting self-esteem, social integration, and overall life satisfaction.
- **Health Outcomes**: Addressing mental health needs and providing psychosocial support contribute to improved health outcomes, symptom management, and disease self-management in HIV-infected individuals across the continuum of care.

Future Directions and Innovations

Advancements in supportive care and holistic approaches in HIV/AIDS focus on innovative interventions, evidence-based practices, and integrated healthcare delivery models to enhance patient-centered care, optimize health outcomes, and reduce health disparities:
- **Telehealth and Digital Interventions**: Integration of telehealth platforms, mobile health applications, and digital therapeutics expands access to mental health services, counseling support, and peer networks for individuals living with HIV/AIDS.
- **Cultural Competency**: Culturally responsive care models and culturally tailored interventions address diverse cultural beliefs, values, and preferences, promoting trust, engagement, and therapeutic alliance in HIV/AIDS care settings.
- **Community Engagement**: Community-based participatory research, community health worker programs, and peer-led initiatives empower local communities, promote health literacy, and advocate for equitable access to supportive care resources.

Conclusion

Supportive care and holistic approaches are essential pillars of HIV/AIDS management, encompassing nutritional support, mental health services, and counseling interventions tailored to address the diverse needs of individuals affected by

HIV infection. Understanding the principles, strategies, and impact of supportive care interventions enhances healthcare providers' capacity to deliver comprehensive, patient-centered care, optimize treatment outcomes, and promote holistic well-being across the lifespan of individuals living with HIV/AIDS. Integrated approaches that integrate medical, psychosocial, and community-based support contribute to achieving sustained viral suppression, improving quality of life, and advancing health equity in the global response to HIV/AIDS.

CHAPTER 7: PREVENTION AND PUBLIC HEALTH STRATEGIES

Primary Prevention of HIV/AIDS

Primary prevention strategies play a pivotal role in reducing the incidence and transmission of Human Immunodeficiency Virus (HIV) infection, emphasizing education, behavioral interventions, and biomedical approaches to promote safer practices and reduce HIV transmission risks. This section explores the principles, strategies, and specific interventions within primary prevention efforts, focusing on education and awareness programs, safer sex practices, and pre-exposure prophylaxis (PrEP).

Introduction to Primary Prevention

Primary prevention aims to prevent initial HIV infection and transmission among individuals at risk through targeted interventions addressing behavioral, biomedical, and structural factors influencing HIV vulnerability. Effective primary prevention strategies are integral to comprehensive HIV/AIDS control efforts, promoting health equity, and reducing the global burden of HIV infection.

Principles of Primary Prevention

Primary prevention strategies are guided by key principles that

include:
- **Behavioral Change**: Promoting informed decision-making, empowering individuals to adopt safer behaviors, and reducing HIV transmission risks through education, counseling, and community engagement.
- **Biomedical Interventions**: Implementing evidence-based biomedical interventions (e.g., PrEP, condoms) to reduce HIV acquisition risks and enhance protection among at-risk populations.
- **Structural Interventions**: Addressing social determinants of health (e.g., stigma, discrimination, access to healthcare) to create supportive environments conducive to HIV prevention and care.

Education and Awareness Programs

Education and awareness programs are foundational components of primary prevention, providing essential knowledge, promoting risk reduction behaviors, and challenging misconceptions about HIV/AIDS transmission, prevention, and stigma.

Key Components of Education and Awareness Programs
- **HIV Transmission Dynamics**: Understanding modes of HIV transmission (e.g., sexual contact, sharing needles, perinatal transmission) and dispelling myths and misconceptions about routes of transmission.
- **Condom Use and Safer Sex Practices**: Promoting consistent and correct condom use during sexual activity, discussing negotiation skills, and advocating for mutual monogamy or sexual abstinence among at-risk individuals.
- **Harm Reduction Strategies**: Providing education on harm reduction approaches for individuals who inject drugs (e.g., needle exchange programs, opioid substitution therapy) to reduce risks of HIV

transmission and overdose.
- **HIV Testing and Counseling**: Promoting routine HIV testing, voluntary counseling and testing (VCT) services, and linkage to care for early diagnosis, treatment initiation, and prevention of onward transmission.

Target Populations
- **General Population**: Comprehensive education programs target the general public to increase awareness, knowledge, and understanding of HIV/AIDS prevention strategies and promote supportive attitudes towards affected individuals.
- **Key Populations**: Tailored education initiatives focus on key populations at higher risk of HIV infection (e.g., men who have sex with men [MSM], transgender individuals, sex workers, people who inject drugs [PWID], and incarcerated populations), addressing specific cultural, social, and structural barriers to prevention.
- **Youth and Adolescents**: Youth-specific education programs emphasize age-appropriate sexual health education, risk reduction strategies, and skills-building to empower young people in making informed decisions about their sexual health.

Safer Sex Practices

Safer sex practices are fundamental in reducing HIV transmission risks and preventing sexually transmitted infections (STIs) among sexually active individuals. Effective promotion of safer sex practices includes comprehensive education, access to condoms, and support for behavior change strategies.

Components of Safer Sex Practices
- **Condom Use**: Advocating for consistent and correct condom use during vaginal, anal, and oral sexual

activities to reduce the risk of HIV transmission and other STIs.

- **Dual Protection**: Encouraging dual protection methods (e.g., condoms and PrEP) for individuals at high risk of HIV infection to maximize prevention efficacy and reduce transmission risks.
- **Negotiation Skills**: Building skills in communication, negotiation, and assertiveness to facilitate discussions about safer sex practices, condom use, and sexual health with partners.
- **Regular STI Testing**: Promoting regular screening and treatment for STIs, including HIV, syphilis, gonorrhea, and chlamydia, to prevent complications, reduce transmission risks, and promote sexual health.

Behavioral Interventions

- **Behavioral Counseling**: Providing individual or group counseling sessions that focus on risk reduction strategies, decision-making skills, and goal-setting to support sustained adherence to safer sex practices.
- **Sexual Health Promotion**: Integrating sexual health promotion into healthcare settings, community-based organizations, and educational institutions to normalize discussions about sexual health, reduce stigma, and empower individuals to take proactive steps in protecting their health.

Pre-Exposure Prophylaxis (PrEP)

Pre-exposure prophylaxis (PrEP) represents a biomedical intervention that offers effective HIV prevention for individuals at substantial risk of HIV infection. PrEP involves the use of antiretroviral medications by HIV-negative individuals to prevent acquisition of the virus before potential exposure.

Mechanism of PrEP

- **Antiretroviral Medications**: PrEP regimens typically consist of daily oral dosing of tenofovir disoproxil

fumarate (TDF) and emtricitabine (FTC) or a combination of tenofovir alafenamide (TAF) and emtricitabine, which block HIV replication within target cells, preventing establishment of systemic infection.
- **Mode of Action**: PrEP medications achieve protective drug concentrations in mucosal tissues (e.g., genital tract, rectal mucosa) and systemic circulation, reducing the risk of HIV acquisition if exposure occurs.

Indications and Eligibility for PrEP
- **High-Risk Individuals**: PrEP is recommended for individuals at substantial risk of HIV infection, including MSM, transgender individuals, heterosexual individuals with multiple partners, individuals who inject drugs, and serodiscordant couples (where one partner is HIV-positive and the other is HIV-negative).
- **Clinical Guidelines**: Eligibility for PrEP is determined based on individual risk assessment, HIV testing, renal function assessment, and adherence to PrEP medication regimens as outlined in national and international clinical guidelines.

Implementation and Adherence
- **Access and Affordability**: Ensuring equitable access to PrEP through healthcare systems, community clinics, and public health programs to reach populations at highest risk of HIV infection, including uninsured or underinsured individuals.
- **Adherence Support**: Implementation of adherence support strategies (e.g., medication adherence counseling, reminder tools, peer support programs) to enhance PrEP uptake, persistence, and effectiveness in preventing HIV acquisition.

Monitoring and Follow-Up
- **HIV Testing and STI Screening**: Regular HIV testing

(e.g., every 3 months) and screening for other STIs are recommended as part of PrEP monitoring to ensure early detection of HIV infection, assess medication adherence, and optimize overall sexual health.

Public Health Impact
- **Reduction in HIV Incidence**: PrEP implementation contributes to significant reductions in HIV incidence among at-risk populations, supporting public health efforts to achieve HIV epidemic control and eliminate new HIV infections.

Integration of Primary Prevention Strategies

Integration of education and awareness programs, promotion of safer sex practices, and expanded access to PrEP are essential components of comprehensive primary prevention strategies, synergistically addressing behavioral, biomedical, and structural determinants of HIV vulnerability:

- **Multifaceted Approaches**: Comprehensive primary prevention approaches combine behavioral interventions, biomedical strategies, and structural interventions to maximize prevention impact, reduce transmission risks, and promote population-level health outcomes.
- **Community Engagement**: Engaging communities, stakeholders, and key populations in the design, implementation, and evaluation of primary prevention initiatives fosters trust, participation, and sustainability of HIV/AIDS prevention efforts.

Challenges and Future Directions
- **Stigma and Discrimination**: Addressing stigma and discrimination associated with HIV/AIDS remains a barrier to effective prevention efforts, requiring targeted interventions to promote inclusivity, respect human rights, and reduce social barriers to healthcare access.

- **Health Disparities**: Disparities in access to HIV prevention services, including PrEP, among marginalized populations (e.g., racial and ethnic minorities, LGBTQ+ individuals, socioeconomically disadvantaged groups) necessitate health equity-focused approaches to ensure equitable access and reduce disparities in HIV incidence.
- **Research and Innovation**: Ongoing research and innovation in HIV prevention technologies, including long-acting PrEP formulations, HIV vaccines, and novel biomedical interventions, advance the field towards sustainable solutions for achieving global HIV/AIDS epidemic control and elimination goals.

Conclusion

Primary prevention strategies are critical in the global response to HIV/AIDS, emphasizing education, behavioral interventions, and biomedical approaches to reduce HIV transmission risks, promote safer practices, and empower individuals and communities in HIV prevention efforts. Understanding the principles, strategies, and impact of primary prevention interventions enhances healthcare providers' capacity to deliver effective, evidence-based HIV prevention services, mitigate transmission risks, and promote health equity worldwide. Integrated approaches that combine education, behavioral interventions, and biomedical advancements contribute to achieving sustained reductions in HIV incidence, improving public health outcomes, and advancing towards the goal of ending the HIV/AIDS epidemic.

Secondary Prevention of HIV/AIDS

Secondary prevention strategies focus on early detection, timely intervention, and effective management of Human Immunodeficiency Virus (HIV) infection among individuals already diagnosed with the virus. These strategies aim to reduce HIV-related morbidity and mortality, prevent onward transmission, and optimize health outcomes through early diagnosis, prompt initiation of antiretroviral therapy (ART), and implementation of harm reduction strategies. This section explores the principles, components, and clinical implications of secondary prevention efforts in HIV/AIDS care.

Introduction to Secondary Prevention

Secondary prevention in HIV/AIDS care encompasses a continuum of interventions aimed at individuals living with HIV infection, emphasizing proactive healthcare strategies to prevent disease progression, reduce transmission risks, and enhance overall well-being. Effective secondary prevention strategies are essential components of comprehensive HIV/AIDS management, promoting early diagnosis, linkage to care, and adherence to treatment to achieve viral suppression and improve clinical outcomes.

Principles of Secondary Prevention

Secondary prevention strategies are guided by principles that include:

- **Early Diagnosis**: Facilitating timely HIV testing, diagnosis, and linkage to care to ensure early initiation of antiretroviral therapy (ART) and prevent delays in treatment initiation.
- **Optimal Treatment Adherence**: Promoting sustained adherence to ART regimens to achieve and maintain viral suppression, reduce HIV transmission risks, and prevent development of antiretroviral resistance.
- **Risk Reduction Strategies**: Implementing harm reduction approaches (e.g., needle exchange programs, opioid substitution therapy) to mitigate risks of secondary infections, substance use-related complications, and comorbidities among individuals living with HIV/AIDS.

Early Diagnosis and Treatment

Early diagnosis and prompt initiation of antiretroviral therapy (ART) are cornerstone components of secondary prevention, promoting clinical outcomes, reducing transmission risks, and improving quality of life for individuals living with HIV infection.

Importance of Early Diagnosis

- **Clinical Benefits**: Early diagnosis facilitates timely access to HIV care and treatment, reduces risks of HIV-related morbidity and mortality, and improves long-term health outcomes.
- **Public Health Impact**: Early detection of HIV infection enables implementation of prevention strategies (e.g., partner notification, behavioral counseling) to reduce onward transmission risks and prevent new HIV infections.

Strategies for Early Diagnosis

- **Routine HIV Testing**: Implementing routine HIV testing recommendations in healthcare settings, community-based organizations, and outreach programs to increase awareness, promote testing uptake, and identify undiagnosed individuals living with HIV infection.
- **Opt-Out Testing**: Offering opt-out HIV testing as part of routine medical care, prenatal care, and sexually transmitted infection (STI) screening to normalize testing, reduce stigma, and improve detection of HIV infection among diverse populations.
- **Targeted Testing**: Targeting populations at higher risk of HIV infection (e.g., MSM, transgender individuals, people who inject drugs [PWID], incarcerated populations) with tailored testing initiatives and outreach strategies to enhance case finding and early diagnosis.

Benefits of Early Treatment Initiation

- **Viral Suppression**: Early initiation of ART suppresses HIV viral replication, preserves immune function, and reduces risks of HIV-related complications and progression to acquired immunodeficiency syndrome (AIDS).
- **Transmission Prevention**: Achieving and maintaining viral suppression through ART reduces HIV transmission risks by lowering viral load levels in bodily fluids (e.g., blood, genital secretions), supporting individual health and public health objectives.

Clinical Guidelines and Recommendations

- **ART Initiation Criteria**: National and international clinical guidelines recommend ART initiation for all individuals diagnosed with HIV infection, regardless of CD4 T-cell count, to maximize treatment benefits, improve health outcomes, and reduce transmission risks.
- **Adherence Support**: Providing comprehensive adherence support services (e.g., adherence counseling, reminder tools, peer support programs) to promote sustained medication adherence, minimize treatment interruptions, and optimize ART efficacy.

Harm Reduction Strategies

Harm reduction strategies are essential components of secondary prevention in HIV/AIDS care, addressing substance use-related risks, reducing transmission of HIV and other blood-borne infections, and promoting health equity among marginalized populations.

Principles of Harm Reduction

- **Health-Centered Approach**: Prioritizing individual health and well-being by minimizing harms associated with substance use through evidence-based interventions and compassionate care.

- **Risk Mitigation**: Mitigating risks of HIV transmission, STIs, overdose, and other health complications associated with substance use behaviors among individuals living with HIV/AIDS.
- **Human Rights and Dignity**: Upholding human rights, dignity, and autonomy of individuals affected by HIV/AIDS and substance use disorders through non-coercive, non-judgmental harm reduction interventions.

Components of Harm Reduction Strategies

- **Needle and Syringe Programs (NSP)**: Implementing NSP to provide sterile needles, syringes, and injection equipment to individuals who inject drugs (PWID), reducing risks of HIV transmission, hepatitis C virus (HCV) infection, and other blood-borne pathogens.
- **Opioid Substitution Therapy (OST)**: Offering OST (e.g., methadone, buprenorphine) as a pharmacological intervention to reduce opioid use, minimize withdrawal symptoms, and support safer injection practices among PWID, promoting health and reducing transmission risks.
- **Safer Injection Practices**: Promoting education on safer injection techniques (e.g., sterile equipment use, vein care, disposal of used needles) to reduce risks of skin and soft tissue infections, bloodstream infections, and HIV transmission among PWID.

Integrated Services and Support

- **Integrated Care Models**: Integrating harm reduction services with HIV/AIDS care, STI screening, mental health support, and social services to address complex health needs, enhance treatment engagement, and improve health outcomes among marginalized populations.
- **Peer Support and Outreach**: Engaging peers with lived

experience in harm reduction programs (e.g., peer outreach, peer support groups) to provide education, support, and linkage to care for individuals at risk of or living with HIV/AIDS and substance use disorders.

Public Health Impact

- **Reduction in Transmission Risks**: Effective implementation of harm reduction strategies contributes to reducing HIV transmission risks, preventing new infections, and promoting community health and safety among vulnerable populations.
- **Health Equity**: Addressing health disparities and promoting equity in access to healthcare, prevention services, and supportive resources for individuals affected by HIV/AIDS and substance use disorders, particularly among marginalized and underserved communities.

Integration of Secondary Prevention Strategies

Integration of early diagnosis and treatment initiatives with harm reduction strategies enhances the effectiveness of secondary prevention efforts in HIV/AIDS care, promoting health equity, reducing transmission risks, and improving health outcomes:

- **Comprehensive Care Continuum**: Coordinated implementation of secondary prevention strategies across healthcare settings, community-based organizations, and public health programs supports seamless transitions in HIV care, promotes retention in care, and optimizes treatment adherence.
- **Collaborative Partnerships**: Collaborative partnerships between healthcare providers, community organizations, peer networks, and policymakers facilitate interdisciplinary approaches to addressing complex health needs, supporting health promotion, and advancing HIV/AIDS prevention goals.

Challenges and Future Directions

- **Stigma and Discrimination**: Addressing stigma associated with HIV/AIDS and substance use remains a barrier to accessing and utilizing harm reduction services, necessitating stigma reduction interventions, advocacy efforts, and community engagement strategies.
- **Access to Services**: Ensuring equitable access to HIV testing, ART, harm reduction programs, and supportive services for marginalized populations, including racial and ethnic minorities, LGBTQ+ individuals, and socioeconomically disadvantaged groups, requires targeted interventions and resource allocation.
- **Research and Innovation**: Continued research and innovation in secondary prevention strategies, including novel biomedical interventions, digital health technologies, and implementation science approaches, advance evidence-based practices, and inform policy development to optimize HIV/AIDS care and prevention efforts.

Conclusion

Secondary prevention strategies are critical components of comprehensive HIV/AIDS management, emphasizing early diagnosis, timely intervention, and effective management of HIV infection to reduce transmission risks, improve health outcomes, and promote health equity. Understanding the principles, components, and clinical implications of secondary prevention interventions enhances healthcare providers' capacity to deliver integrated, patient-centered care, mitigate HIV-related morbidity and mortality, and advance towards achieving global HIV/AIDS epidemic control goals. Integrated approaches that combine early diagnosis, treatment initiation, and harm reduction strategies support sustainable reductions in HIV transmission, enhance quality of life, and promote holistic well-being among individuals living with HIV/AIDS worldwide.

Tertiary Prevention and Supportive Care in HIV/AIDS

Tertiary prevention and supportive care in the context of HIV/AIDS aim to optimize health outcomes, enhance quality of life, and mitigate complications among individuals living with Human Immunodeficiency Virus (HIV) infection. This section explores the principles, components, and clinical implications of tertiary prevention strategies and supportive care interventions in HIV/AIDS management.

Introduction to Tertiary Prevention and Supportive Care

Tertiary prevention focuses on minimizing the impact of established HIV infection, managing complications, and promoting health maintenance and rehabilitation. Supportive care encompasses a range of interventions aimed at addressing physical, psychological, social, and emotional needs of individuals living with HIV/AIDS, promoting holistic well-being and improving overall quality of life.

Principles of Tertiary Prevention

Tertiary prevention strategies in HIV/AIDS care are guided by principles that include:

- **Multidisciplinary Approach**: Collaborative involvement of healthcare providers, specialists, allied health professionals, and community resources to address complex health needs and optimize comprehensive care delivery.
- **Chronic Disease Management**: Integration of chronic disease management principles to monitor disease progression, manage complications, and promote adherence to treatment and supportive care interventions.

- **Patient-Centered Care**: Individualized care planning, shared decision-making, and patient empowerment to address diverse health concerns, preferences, and goals of individuals living with HIV/AIDS.

Components of Tertiary Prevention and Supportive Care

Tertiary prevention and supportive care interventions encompass a continuum of services and interventions aimed at enhancing health outcomes, promoting adherence to treatment, and addressing physical, psychological, social, and emotional needs of individuals affected by HIV/AIDS:

Medical Management and Disease Monitoring

- **Comprehensive HIV Care**: Provision of ongoing HIV medical care, including routine monitoring of HIV viral load, CD4 T-cell count, and clinical assessments to optimize treatment efficacy, monitor disease progression, and detect complications early.
- **Management of Comorbidities**: Screening, prevention, and management of HIV-related comorbidities (e.g., cardiovascular disease, diabetes, renal impairment) and non-AIDS defining conditions to mitigate risks and improve overall health outcomes.
- **Antiretroviral Therapy (ART)**: Optimization of ART regimens based on individual treatment response, viral resistance testing, and adherence support strategies to achieve and maintain viral suppression, reduce transmission risks, and preserve immune function.

Psychosocial Support and Mental Health Services

- **Behavioral Health Counseling**: Provision of individual, group, or family counseling services to address psychological and emotional challenges associated with HIV/AIDS diagnosis, treatment adherence, stigma, and mental health disorders (e.g., depression, anxiety).

- **Peer Support Programs**: Engagement of peers with lived experience in HIV/AIDS care (e.g., peer navigation, support groups) to provide emotional support, share coping strategies, and foster social connections among individuals living with HIV/AIDS.
- **Stigma Reduction Interventions**: Implementation of stigma reduction initiatives (e.g., education, advocacy, community outreach) to combat HIV-related stigma, promote social inclusion, and enhance resilience among affected individuals and communities.

Palliative and End-of-Life Care

- **Pain and Symptom Management**: Provision of palliative care services to alleviate physical symptoms (e.g., pain, fatigue, nausea) associated with advanced HIV disease or treatment side effects, enhancing comfort and quality of life.
- **Advance Care Planning**: Facilitation of discussions on advance care planning, end-of-life preferences, and supportive care options to empower individuals living with HIV/AIDS in making informed decisions about their healthcare preferences and goals.
- **Bereavement Support**: Provision of bereavement counseling and support services to individuals and families affected by HIV/AIDS-related loss, promoting emotional healing, and coping with grief.

Nutritional Support and Wellness Programs

- **Dietary Counseling**: Provision of nutritional assessment, counseling, and education to optimize dietary intake, manage nutritional deficiencies, and support overall health and immune function in individuals living with HIV/AIDS.
- **Exercise and Wellness Programs**: Promotion of physical activity, wellness initiatives, and lifestyle modifications to enhance cardiovascular health,

mitigate metabolic complications, and improve quality of life among individuals affected by HIV/AIDS.
- **Substance Use Disorders Management**: Integration of substance use disorder screening, treatment, and harm reduction strategies to address concurrent substance use disorders, reduce risks of HIV transmission, and promote health and recovery.

Social Services and Community Resources
- **Case Management Services**: Coordination of social services (e.g., housing assistance, financial counseling, legal advocacy) to address social determinants of health, improve access to care, and promote stability and well-being among individuals living with HIV/AIDS.
- **Community Engagement**: Collaboration with community-based organizations, peer networks, and advocacy groups to promote health equity, raise awareness about HIV/AIDS prevention and care, and address systemic barriers affecting marginalized populations.
- **Health Education and Empowerment**: Provision of health education programs, skills-building workshops, and empowerment initiatives to enhance health literacy, promote self-management skills, and foster resilience among individuals living with HIV/AIDS.

Integration of Tertiary Prevention and Supportive Care

Integration of tertiary prevention and supportive care interventions in HIV/AIDS management optimizes health outcomes, enhances quality of life, and addresses holistic health needs of individuals living with HIV/AIDS:
- **Continuum of Care**: Seamless integration of medical management, psychosocial support, palliative care, and wellness services across healthcare settings, community-based organizations, and public health

programs to support sustained engagement in HIV care.

- **Patient-Centered Approach**: Collaborative care planning, patient education, and shared decision-making processes that prioritize individual preferences, needs, and goals to promote empowerment, autonomy, and self-efficacy in HIV/AIDS care.

Challenges and Future Directions

- **Healthcare Access and Equity**: Addressing disparities in access to HIV/AIDS care, supportive services, and resources among underserved populations (e.g., racial and ethnic minorities, LGBTQ+ communities, socioeconomically disadvantaged groups) through targeted interventions and policy initiatives.

- **Multimorbidity and Aging**: Managing complexities associated with multimorbidity, aging-related health concerns, and long-term HIV/AIDS survivorship through integrated care models, geriatric assessments, and age-appropriate health promotion strategies.

- **Research and Innovation**: Advancing research in supportive care interventions, palliative care models, and innovative therapies to address evolving healthcare needs, enhance treatment outcomes, and improve quality of life for individuals living with HIV/AIDS.

Conclusion

Tertiary prevention and supportive care interventions are integral components of comprehensive HIV/AIDS management, focusing on optimizing health outcomes, promoting quality of life, and addressing diverse health needs of individuals living with HIV infection. Understanding the principles, components, and clinical implications of tertiary prevention strategies enhances healthcare providers' capacity to deliver patient-centered care, support long-term health and well-being, and advance towards achieving individual and public health goals in HIV/AIDS care. Integrated approaches that prioritize holistic care, address psychosocial needs, and promote resilience contribute to enhancing health equity, reducing HIV-related disparities, and improving overall quality of life for individuals affected by HIV/AIDS globally.

CHAPTER 8: SOCIETAL IMPACTS AND ETHICAL CONSIDERATIONS

Stigma and Discrimination in HIV/AIDS

Stigma and discrimination remain significant barriers in the global response to HIV/AIDS, affecting individuals living with HIV, their families, and communities. This section examines the pervasive nature of stigma, its detrimental effects on health outcomes and well-being, and strategies for combating stigma and promoting social inclusion.

Introduction to Stigma and Discrimination

Stigma is a social process that devalues individuals or groups based on perceived differences from societal norms or expectations. Discrimination, on the other hand, involves actions that result in unequal treatment or denial of rights to individuals or groups due to these perceived differences. In the context of HIV/AIDS, stigma and discrimination have profound implications, exacerbating health disparities and hindering efforts to prevent new infections and provide equitable care and support.

Historical Context of HIV/AIDS Stigma

The stigma associated with HIV/AIDS has deep historical roots, shaped by fear, misinformation, and moral judgments. During the early years of the epidemic, HIV/AIDS was often perceived as a "gay disease" or a punishment for perceived immoral behavior, leading to widespread stigma, discrimination, and social exclusion. These negative attitudes persisted despite advancements in scientific understanding and public health education.

Forms and Manifestations of Stigma

Stigma related to HIV/AIDS manifests in various forms, including:

- **Social Stigma**: Negative attitudes, prejudice, and stereotypes towards individuals living with HIV/AIDS within communities and broader society.
- **Structural Stigma**: Discriminatory policies, laws, and institutional practices that perpetuate inequalities and restrict access to healthcare, employment, housing, and other essential services for individuals affected by HIV/AIDS.
- **Self-Stigma**: Internalized shame, guilt, and self-blame experienced by individuals living with HIV/AIDS as a result of societal stigma, impacting self-esteem, mental health, and healthcare-seeking behaviors.
- **Intersectional Stigma**: Overlapping stigmas related to race, ethnicity, gender identity, sexual orientation, socioeconomic status, and other marginalized identities, compounding the experiences of discrimination and exclusion.

Impact of Stigma and Discrimination

The effects of stigma and discrimination on individuals and communities affected by HIV/AIDS are profound and wide-ranging:

- **Health Outcomes**: Stigma contributes to delayed HIV testing, diagnosis, and linkage to care, resulting in poorer health outcomes, increased HIV transmission rates, and reduced adherence to antiretroviral therapy

(ART).
- **Psychosocial Well-being**: Stigma undermines mental health, leading to anxiety, depression, social isolation, and diminished quality of life among individuals living with HIV/AIDS and their families.
- **Economic Consequences**: Discrimination in employment and housing opportunities limits economic stability and exacerbates poverty among individuals affected by HIV/AIDS, perpetuating cycles of vulnerability and exclusion.
- **Human Rights Violations**: Violations of human rights, including denial of healthcare, education, and legal protections, perpetuate social injustices and hinder efforts to achieve health equity and social justice.

Addressing Stigma and Discrimination

Combatting stigma and discrimination in the context of HIV/AIDS requires multifaceted approaches at individual, community, institutional, and policy levels:

Education and Awareness

- **Public Health Campaigns**: Implementing comprehensive education campaigns to dispel myths, challenge stereotypes, and promote accurate information about HIV transmission, prevention, and treatment.
- **Community Engagement**: Engaging affected communities, healthcare providers, and stakeholders in dialogue and advocacy efforts to raise awareness, reduce stigma, and promote solidarity and support for individuals living with HIV/AIDS.

Legal and Policy Reforms

- **Anti-Discrimination Laws**: Advocating for and enforcing laws that protect the rights of individuals living with HIV/AIDS against discrimination in healthcare, employment, housing, education, and

other domains.
- **Healthcare Access**: Ensuring equitable access to healthcare services, including HIV testing, treatment, and supportive care, through policy initiatives that address systemic barriers and promote health equity.

Empowerment and Support
- **Peer Support Programs**: Establishing peer-led support groups and networks to provide emotional support, share experiences, and empower individuals living with HIV/AIDS to advocate for their rights and access healthcare services.
- **Counseling and Mental Health Services**: Integrating psychosocial support, counseling, and mental health services into HIV/AIDS care to address stigma-related stressors, promote resilience, and enhance overall well-being.

Media and Communications
- **Responsible Reporting**: Promoting responsible media reporting and portrayal of HIV/AIDS issues to reduce sensationalism, combat stereotypes, and promote empathy and understanding in public discourse.
- **Digital Advocacy**: Utilizing digital platforms and social media to amplify voices of individuals living with HIV/AIDS, share personal stories, and foster community support and solidarity.

Global Perspectives and Challenges

Addressing stigma and discrimination in HIV/AIDS requires global collaboration, cultural sensitivity, and sustained advocacy efforts:
- **Cultural Context**: Recognizing cultural beliefs, norms, and practices that influence perceptions of HIV/AIDS and stigma within diverse communities, tailoring interventions to respect cultural values and promote

inclusivity.
- **Intersectional Approaches**: Adopting intersectional approaches that address overlapping stigmas and inequalities based on race, ethnicity, gender identity, sexual orientation, and socioeconomic status to promote health equity and social justice.
- **Policy Implementation**: Overcoming barriers to policy implementation, resource allocation, and enforcement of anti-discrimination laws to ensure meaningful protections and rights for individuals living with HIV/AIDS worldwide.

Conclusion

Stigma and discrimination remain formidable challenges in the global response to HIV/AIDS, undermining efforts to achieve equitable access to healthcare, promote health outcomes, and ensure social justice for affected individuals and communities. Addressing stigma requires coordinated efforts across multiple sectors, including education, policy reform, healthcare delivery, and community engagement, to challenge stereotypes, empower individuals, and foster inclusive environments. By advancing stigma reduction initiatives, promoting empathy, and protecting human rights, we can create a world where individuals living with HIV/AIDS are treated with dignity, respect, and compassion, and where health equity and social justice prevail.

Legal and Human Rights Issues in HIV/AIDS

The legal and human rights dimensions of HIV/AIDS encompass a complex interplay of laws, policies, social attitudes, and systemic barriers that impact the lives of individuals living with HIV/AIDS, their families, and communities. This section examines the legal frameworks, human rights violations, stigma, discrimination, and advocacy efforts shaping the response to HIV/AIDS globally.

Legal Frameworks and Human Rights Protections

Legal frameworks play a pivotal role in safeguarding the rights and dignity of individuals affected by HIV/AIDS, ensuring access to healthcare, prevention services, and protection against discrimination. Key aspects include:

International Human Rights Standards

- **Universal Declaration of Human Rights**: Affirms the right to health, non-discrimination, privacy, and dignity, forming the basis for human rights protections for individuals living with HIV/AIDS.
- **International Covenant on Civil and Political Rights (ICCPR)**: Guarantees civil and political rights, including the right to privacy, non-discrimination, and access to justice, essential for upholding the rights of individuals affected by HIV/AIDS.
- **International Covenant on Economic, Social, and Cultural Rights (ICESCR)**: Recognizes the right to health, including access to essential medicines and healthcare services, critical for addressing HIV/AIDS-related health disparities and promoting health equity.

National Legislation and Policies

- **Anti-Discrimination Laws**: Legislative measures prohibiting discrimination based on HIV status in employment, healthcare, education, housing, and other domains, essential for protecting the rights of individuals living with HIV/AIDS.
- **Healthcare Access Laws**: Legislation ensuring equitable access to HIV testing, treatment, and supportive care services, addressing systemic barriers and promoting health equity for marginalized populations.
- **Privacy and Confidentiality Protections**: Legal safeguards protecting the confidentiality of HIV-related information, crucial for reducing stigma,

promoting HIV testing uptake, and ensuring privacy rights for individuals living with HIV/AIDS.

Human Rights Violations and Challenges

Despite legal protections and international commitments, individuals affected by HIV/AIDS continue to face human rights violations, stigma, and discrimination:

Stigma and Discrimination

- **Social Stigma**: Negative attitudes, stereotypes, and prejudice towards individuals living with HIV/AIDS within communities and broader society, contributing to social exclusion, isolation, and diminished quality of life.
- **Structural Discrimination**: Discriminatory policies, laws, and institutional practices that perpetuate inequalities and restrict access to healthcare, employment, housing, and other essential services for individuals affected by HIV/AIDS.
- **Intersectional Stigma**: Overlapping stigmas based on race, ethnicity, gender identity, sexual orientation, and socioeconomic status, compounding experiences of discrimination and exclusion among marginalized populations.

Criminalization of HIV Non-Disclosure and Exposure

- **Laws Criminalizing HIV Non-Disclosure**: Legal statutes imposing criminal penalties for nondisclosure of HIV-positive status or potential exposure, often based on outdated notions of HIV transmission risk and stigma, undermining public health goals and human rights protections.
- **Impact on Public Health**: Criminalization laws deter individuals from accessing HIV testing, treatment, and prevention services, perpetuate fear and stigma, and hinder efforts to promote open communication and prevention strategies.

Access to Justice and Legal Representation

- **Legal Aid Services**: Limited availability of legal aid services and representation for individuals affected by HIV/AIDS, particularly among marginalized populations, hindering access to justice, advocacy for rights, and defense against discrimination.
- **Barriers to Legal Redress**: Systemic barriers such as poverty, lack of legal awareness, stigma, and discrimination within judicial systems that impede access to legal redress and enforcement of human rights protections for individuals living with HIV/AIDS.

Strategies for Legal Empowerment and Advocacy

Addressing legal and human rights issues in HIV/AIDS requires coordinated efforts across multiple sectors and stakeholders:

Legal Reform and Policy Advocacy

- **Repealing Discriminatory Laws**: Advocating for the repeal of laws criminalizing HIV non-disclosure or exposure based on scientific evidence, public health principles, and human rights standards to promote supportive legal environments.
- **Promoting Anti-Discrimination Protections**: Strengthening implementation and enforcement of anti-discrimination laws and policies to protect the rights of individuals living with HIV/AIDS in healthcare, employment, education, and other settings.

Human Rights Education and Awareness

- **Training for Legal Professionals**: Providing training and education for legal professionals, healthcare providers, law enforcement officials, and community advocates on HIV/AIDS-related human rights issues, stigma reduction, and legal empowerment strategies.

- **Community Engagement**: Empowering affected communities through grassroots advocacy, peer support networks, and human rights education initiatives to promote awareness, resilience, and collective action against stigma and discrimination.

Strengthening Health and Legal Systems Integration

- **Integrated Service Delivery**: Enhancing collaboration between health and legal systems to integrate HIV/AIDS care, legal aid services, and advocacy efforts, ensuring holistic support and rights-based approaches for individuals affected by HIV/AIDS.
- **Policy Development**: Participating in policy development processes to advocate for inclusive healthcare policies, access to justice, and comprehensive HIV/AIDS prevention, treatment, and support services aligned with human rights principles.

Global Perspectives and Challenges

Globally, addressing legal and human rights issues in HIV/AIDS requires collective action, political will, and sustained advocacy efforts:

- **International Cooperation**: Strengthening international cooperation, partnerships, and advocacy networks to advance human rights protections, combat stigma, and promote inclusive policies for individuals living with HIV/AIDS worldwide.
- **Health Equity**: Reducing health disparities and promoting health equity through intersectional approaches that address social determinants of health, structural inequalities, and barriers to healthcare access for marginalized populations affected by HIV/AIDS.
- **Research and Innovation**: Advancing research on legal and human rights impacts of HIV/AIDS, evaluating policy interventions, and innovative strategies to

promote legal empowerment, reduce stigma, and protect human rights in HIV/AIDS responses.

Conclusion

Legal and human rights issues are integral to the global response to HIV/AIDS, influencing health outcomes, access to care, and social inclusion for individuals affected by the epidemic. By upholding human rights standards, challenging stigma and discrimination, and advocating for supportive legal environments, we can create inclusive societies where individuals living with HIV/AIDS are empowered, respected, and able to access the healthcare and support services they need. Through collaborative efforts, legal empowerment, and policy advocacy, we can advance towards achieving health equity, promoting social justice, and ending the stigma and discrimination associated with HIV/AIDS globally.

Ethical Challenges in Research and Treatment of HIV/AIDS

Ethical considerations are paramount in the research, prevention, and treatment of HIV/AIDS, ensuring that scientific advancements and healthcare practices uphold principles of beneficence, respect for autonomy, justice, and non-maleficence. This section delves into the ethical complexities, dilemmas, and best practices in HIV/AIDS research and treatment, addressing key issues and frameworks guiding ethical decision-making.

Introduction to Ethical Challenges

Ethical challenges in HIV/AIDS research and treatment encompass a range of issues related to:

- **Informed Consent**: Ensuring voluntary and informed participation of individuals in research studies and clinical trials, respecting autonomy and protecting participants' rights.
- **Equity and Access**: Promoting equitable access to HIV

prevention, treatment, and care services, addressing disparities, and advocating for social justice in healthcare delivery.
- **Stigma and Discrimination**: Addressing stigma and discrimination in research settings, healthcare practices, and public health interventions to promote dignity and respect for individuals affected by HIV/AIDS.
- **Public Health Priorities**: Balancing individual rights with public health priorities, including prevention strategies, treatment access, and ethical allocation of resources.

Ethical Principles in HIV/AIDS Research

Ethical principles guide the conduct of HIV/AIDS research, ensuring scientific rigor, participant safety, and respect for human rights:

Beneficence and Non-Maleficence

- **Beneficence**: Maximizing benefits and minimizing harm to research participants, ensuring that research protocols prioritize participant well-being and contribute to scientific knowledge advancement.
- **Non-Maleficence**: Avoiding harm and minimizing risks associated with research interventions, including potential adverse effects of experimental treatments or preventive measures.

Respect for Autonomy

- **Informed Consent**: Obtaining voluntary and informed consent from research participants, ensuring comprehension of study procedures, potential risks, benefits, and alternatives to participation.
- **Privacy and Confidentiality**: Protecting participants' privacy rights and confidentiality of personal health information, maintaining trust and respect for individuals' autonomy in research settings.

Justice

- **Equitable Access**: Promoting fair distribution of research benefits and burdens across diverse populations, addressing disparities in access to research opportunities and healthcare services.
- **Inclusion and Diversity**: Ensuring representation of diverse populations in research studies, addressing health disparities, and advancing health equity through inclusive research practices.

Ethical Considerations in HIV/AIDS Treatment

Ethical dilemmas in HIV/AIDS treatment encompass issues related to:

- **Antiretroviral Therapy (ART)**: Access, adherence, and equitable distribution of ART medications, ensuring timely initiation, sustained treatment adherence, and management of treatment-related side effects.
- **Resource Allocation**: Ethical decision-making in resource-limited settings, prioritizing allocation of healthcare resources, including medications, diagnostic tests, and supportive care services, based on clinical need and public health impact.
- **End-of-Life Care**: Palliative care, advance care planning, and ethical considerations in decision-making regarding end-of-life preferences, dignity, and quality of life for individuals living with advanced HIV/AIDS.

Ethical Challenges in HIV/AIDS Research

Research with Vulnerable Populations

- **Pregnant Women and Children**: Ethical considerations in conducting research involving pregnant women, infants, and children affected by HIV/AIDS, ensuring protection of minors and maternal health considerations.

- **Key Populations**: Ethical challenges in research involving key populations disproportionately affected by HIV/AIDS, including men who have sex with men, transgender individuals, sex workers, people who inject drugs, and incarcerated populations.

Prevention Trials and Risk Reduction Strategies

- **Pre-Exposure Prophylaxis (PrEP)**: Ethical considerations in PrEP research, including risk assessment, adherence monitoring, and provision of comprehensive prevention services to study participants at increased risk of HIV infection.
- **Vaccine Research**: Ethical dilemmas in HIV vaccine trials, balancing potential benefits of vaccine development with participant safety, informed consent, and risk communication strategies.

Ethical Guidelines and Regulatory Frameworks

Ethical guidelines and regulatory frameworks provide guidance and oversight in HIV/AIDS research and treatment:

- **Declaration of Helsinki**: Principles guiding ethical conduct of medical research involving human participants, emphasizing voluntary informed consent, participant welfare, and scientific integrity.
- **Good Clinical Practice (GCP)**: International standards for designing, conducting, and reporting clinical trials, ensuring ethical conduct, data integrity, and participant safety in HIV/AIDS research studies.
- **National and Institutional Ethics Review Boards**: Oversight and approval of research protocols, ensuring adherence to ethical standards, protection of participant rights, and compliance with regulatory requirements.

Ethical Leadership and Advocacy

Ethical leadership and advocacy are essential in addressing

ethical challenges in HIV/AIDS research and treatment:

- **Community Engagement**: Engaging affected communities, advocacy groups, and stakeholders in ethical decision-making, research planning, and policy development to promote transparency, accountability, and community trust.
- **Research Ethics Training**: Providing education and training for researchers, healthcare providers, and ethics committee members on ethical principles, cultural competence, and best practices in HIV/AIDS research and treatment.
- **Policy Advocacy**: Advocating for policies that uphold human rights, address health disparities, and promote ethical research practices, ensuring equitable access to HIV prevention, treatment, and care services for all individuals affected by HIV/AIDS.

Conclusion

Ethical challenges in HIV/AIDS research and treatment underscore the importance of upholding principles of beneficence, respect for autonomy, justice, and non-maleficence in scientific inquiry, healthcare delivery, and public health interventions. By integrating ethical considerations into research protocols, clinical practice guidelines, and policy initiatives, we can advance towards achieving equitable access to HIV prevention, treatment, and care services, promoting human rights, and fostering inclusive and ethical healthcare practices for individuals affected by HIV/AIDS globally. Ethical leadership, community engagement, and advocacy efforts are crucial in addressing complex ethical dilemmas, advancing health equity, and ensuring dignity and respect for all individuals living with HIV/AIDS.

Vaccine Development for HIV/AIDS

The quest for an effective vaccine against HIV/AIDS has been one of the most challenging endeavors in modern medicine and public health. Unlike many other infectious diseases where successful vaccines have been developed, HIV presents unique scientific and immunological hurdles. This section provides an in-depth analysis of the current landscape, challenges, progress, and future prospects of HIV/AIDS vaccine development.

Introduction to HIV Vaccine Development

HIV (Human Immunodeficiency Virus) is a retrovirus that attacks the immune system, specifically targeting CD4+ T cells, crucial components of the body's defense against infections. Developing a vaccine against HIV poses significant challenges due to the virus's ability to mutate rapidly, its diverse genetic variability (multiple subtypes and recombinant forms), and its ability to establish latent reservoirs in the body.

Scientific Foundation and Immunological Challenges

Virus Diversity and Mutability

- **Genetic Variability**: HIV exists as multiple subtypes (clades) and recombinant forms globally, posing challenges in developing a vaccine that can provide broad protection against diverse strains.
- **Mutational Escape**: HIV's high mutation rate allows it to evade immune responses, particularly through mutations in surface glycoproteins like gp120 and gp41, which are targets for neutralizing antibodies.

Immunological Evasion Strategies

- **Evasion of Neutralizing Antibodies**: HIV shields vulnerable epitopes on its surface, making it difficult for antibodies to bind and neutralize the virus effectively.
- **Cellular Immune Responses**: T-cell mediated immunity, particularly CD8+ cytotoxic T lymphocytes (CTLs), play a crucial role in controlling HIV

replication, but inducing protective CTL responses through vaccination remains a challenge.

Historical Perspectives and Vaccine Strategies

Early Vaccine Trials and Setbacks

- **Phase I and II Trials**: Initial vaccine candidates focused on inducing neutralizing antibodies against gp120 and gp41 proteins but faced limited success due to inadequate immune responses and variability in efficacy across different HIV subtypes.
- **RV144 Trial**: The RV144 Thai trial showed modest efficacy (31.2%) in preventing HIV acquisition, utilizing a prime-boost regimen combining a canarypox vector (ALVAC-HIV) and a recombinant gp120 protein (AIDSVAX).

Current Vaccine Approaches

- **Broadly Neutralizing Antibodies (bNAbs)**: Research focuses on isolating and engineering bNAbs capable of neutralizing diverse HIV strains, either for passive immunization or as templates for vaccine design.
- **Viral Vector Vaccines**: Use of viral vectors (e.g., adenovirus, vesicular stomatitis virus) to deliver HIV antigens and stimulate potent cellular and humoral immune responses.
- **mRNA and DNA Vaccines**: Novel vaccine platforms utilizing mRNA or DNA encoding HIV antigens to induce immune responses, promising for their potential to optimize antigen presentation and immune activation.

Challenges in Vaccine Development

Immunological Hurdles

- **Neutralizing Antibody Evasion**: HIV's ability to shield vulnerable epitopes and mutate rapidly necessitates the development of vaccines capable of inducing

broadly neutralizing antibodies (bNAbs).
- **CD8+ T Cell Induction**: Strategies to elicit robust CD8+ T cell responses capable of controlling HIV replication and reducing viral reservoirs remain a priority.

Clinical and Ethical Considerations

- **Clinical Trial Design**: Conducting large-scale efficacy trials in diverse populations, including individuals at high risk of HIV acquisition, while ensuring safety and ethical standards.
- **Ethical Issues**: Ensuring informed consent, confidentiality, and equitable access to vaccine trials, particularly in resource-limited settings and vulnerable populations.

Recent Advances and Future Directions

Advances in Immunogen Design

- **Structural Biology**: Understanding HIV envelope glycoprotein structure and antigen presentation to design immunogens capable of eliciting broadly neutralizing antibodies.
- **Vaccine Adjuvants**: Development of novel adjuvants to enhance immune responses and durability of vaccine-induced protection against HIV.

Collaborative Efforts and Global Initiatives

- **International Collaboration**: Partnership between governments, research institutions, pharmaceutical companies, and global health organizations (e.g., HIV Vaccine Trials Network, International AIDS Vaccine Initiative) to accelerate vaccine development and access.
- **Funding and Investment**: Continued funding and investment in basic research, preclinical studies, and clinical trials to support promising vaccine candidates and innovative approaches.

Conclusion

Developing an effective vaccine against HIV/AIDS remains a formidable scientific and public health challenge, requiring innovative strategies, collaborative efforts, and sustained investment. While progress has been made in understanding HIV immunology and advancing vaccine candidates, significant hurdles remain, including viral diversity, immunological evasion mechanisms, and ethical considerations in research. By leveraging scientific advances, harnessing global partnerships, and prioritizing equitable access to vaccines, the goal of achieving an HIV vaccine that can prevent new infections and contribute to ending the HIV/AIDS pandemic remains within reach. Ethical leadership, community engagement, and commitment to scientific rigor will be crucial in overcoming challenges and advancing towards a world free from HIV/AIDS.

Cure Research for HIV/AIDS

Research toward finding a cure for HIV/AIDS represents a significant frontier in medical science, aiming to achieve sustained virologic remission or eradication of the virus from the body. This section delves into the current landscape, challenges, promising approaches, and ethical considerations in HIV/AIDS cure research.

Introduction to Cure Research

HIV/AIDS cure research focuses on achieving a functional cure (long-term control of HIV replication in the absence of antiretroviral therapy) or a sterilizing cure (complete eradication of HIV from the body). Unlike conventional antiretroviral therapy (ART) that suppresses viral replication, a cure aims to eliminate latent HIV reservoirs, prevent viral rebound upon treatment interruption, and restore immune function.

Scientific Foundations and Challenges

Latent HIV Reservoirs

- **Reservoir Persistence**: HIV establishes latent reservoirs in long-lived CD4+ T cells, macrophages, and other immune cells, remaining dormant and evading immune surveillance and antiretroviral drugs.
- **Viral Rebound**: Interruption of ART often leads to viral rebound due to reactivation of latent HIV reservoirs, highlighting the challenge of achieving sustained virologic remission or cure.

Immunological and Virological Barriers

- **Immune Evasion**: HIV's ability to evade immune responses, including cytotoxic T lymphocytes (CTLs) and neutralizing antibodies, complicates efforts to eliminate infected cells and achieve immune control.
- **Viral Diversity**: Genetic variability and quasispecies formation within HIV populations necessitate approaches capable of targeting diverse viral strains and escape mutants.

Current Approaches to Cure Research

Shock and Kill Strategies

- **Latency-Reversing Agents (LRAs)**: Compounds that activate latent HIV reservoirs, facilitating viral gene expression and rendering infected cells susceptible to immune clearance or cytopathic effects.
- **Immune Modulation**: Strategies to enhance HIV-specific immune responses, including therapeutic vaccines, checkpoint inhibitors, and immune checkpoint blockade, to target and eliminate infected cells.

Gene Therapy and Genome Editing

- **CRISPR/Cas9**: Genome editing technologies to target and excise HIV proviral DNA from infected cells, potentially achieving functional or sterilizing cure

outcomes.
- **Stem Cell Transplantation**: Use of hematopoietic stem cell transplantation (HSCT) with CCR5 Δ32 donor cells, which confer resistance to HIV infection, as demonstrated in the Berlin Patient and other case studies.

Challenges in Cure Research

Latent Reservoirs and Viral Persistence

- **Quantification and Localization**: Challenges in accurately quantifying latent reservoirs, identifying sanctuary sites, and developing therapies that can effectively target and eliminate infected cells throughout the body.
- **Safety and Long-Term Durability**: Ensuring safety of curative interventions, minimizing off-target effects, and achieving durable viral suppression or eradication without compromising immune function.

Clinical Trial Design and Ethics

- **Participant Recruitment**: Inclusion of diverse populations, including individuals with varying HIV subtypes, treatment histories, and comorbidities, in clinical trials evaluating cure strategies.
- **Ethical Considerations**: Informed consent, risk-benefit assessment, and provision of alternative treatment options for participants undergoing experimental cure interventions, particularly in early-phase trials.

Emerging Technologies and Future Directions

Artificial Intelligence and Predictive Modeling

- **Machine Learning**: Utilization of artificial intelligence and predictive modeling to identify optimal combinations of therapeutic agents, personalize treatment regimens, and predict treatment outcomes in cure research.

Collaborative Efforts and Global Initiatives

- **International Consortia**: Collaboration between researchers, healthcare providers, pharmaceutical companies, and community stakeholders through initiatives like the International AIDS Society's Towards an HIV Cure initiative to accelerate research and clinical trials.
- **Funding and Investment**: Continued funding support and investment in basic science, translational research, and clinical trials to advance promising cure strategies and innovations in HIV/AIDS cure research.

Conclusion

Achieving a cure for HIV/AIDS represents a transformative goal in global health, requiring innovative approaches, interdisciplinary collaboration, and sustained investment in research and development. While significant progress has been made in understanding viral persistence, immune evasion mechanisms, and therapeutic interventions, challenges remain in translating scientific discoveries into safe, effective, and scalable cure strategies. By leveraging cutting-edge technologies, enhancing global partnerships, and prioritizing ethical standards in research and clinical practice, the pursuit of an HIV cure holds promise for transforming the lives of individuals living with HIV/AIDS and contributing to the end of the HIV/AIDS pandemic.

Advances in Treatment Strategies for HIV/AIDS

Advances in treatment strategies for HIV/AIDS have revolutionized the management of the virus, significantly improving patient outcomes, reducing mortality rates, and enhancing quality of life. This section explores the evolution of treatment approaches, current therapeutic innovations, challenges, and future directions in HIV/AIDS treatment strategies.

Evolution of HIV/AIDS Treatment

Early Antiretroviral Therapy (ART)

- **Monotherapy and Dual Therapy**: Initial treatments with monotherapy (e.g., zidovudine) and dual therapy (e.g., zidovudine plus lamivudine) aimed at suppressing viral replication and delaying disease progression.
- **Introduction of Highly Active Antiretroviral Therapy (HAART)**: Combination therapy with three or more drugs, including protease inhibitors (PIs), nucleoside reverse transcriptase inhibitors (NRTIs), non-nucleoside reverse transcriptase inhibitors (NNRTIs), and integrase strand transfer inhibitors (INSTIs), revolutionized HIV/AIDS treatment in the mid-1990s.

Standard of Care and Treatment Guidelines

- **Antiretroviral Therapy (ART)**: Guidelines recommend early initiation of ART regardless of CD4 count to achieve viral suppression, preserve immune function, and reduce transmission risk.
- **Individualized Treatment Regimens**: Tailoring ART regimens based on viral load, drug resistance profiles, comorbidities, and patient preferences to optimize efficacy, adherence, and tolerability.

Current Treatment Strategies

Antiretroviral Drug Classes

- **Nucleoside/Nucleotide Reverse Transcriptase Inhibitors (NRTIs/NtRTIs)**: Backbone of most ART regimens, inhibiting viral reverse transcriptase enzyme to prevent viral DNA synthesis.
- **Integrase Strand Transfer Inhibitors (INSTIs)**: Potent inhibitors of HIV integrase enzyme, blocking

integration of viral DNA into host cell genome.

- **Protease Inhibitors (PIs)**: Block protease enzyme, essential for viral maturation, effectively reducing viral replication.
- **Non-Nucleoside Reverse Transcriptase Inhibitors (NNRTIs)**: Bind to and inhibit viral reverse transcriptase enzyme, preventing viral RNA to DNA conversion.

Fixed-Dose Combination Therapies

- **Single Tablet Regimens (STRs)**: Simplified ART regimens combining multiple antiretroviral drugs into a single pill, enhancing adherence, convenience, and treatment outcomes.
- **Long-Acting Formulations**: Extended-release injectable formulations (e.g., cabotegravir/rilpivirine) administered monthly or every two months, providing alternative options for individuals preferring injectable therapies.

Therapeutic Innovations and Strategies

Treatment Optimization

- **Adherence Support**: Behavioral interventions, mobile health technologies, and adherence counseling to enhance treatment adherence and retention in care.
- **Viral Load Monitoring**: Routine monitoring of HIV viral load to assess treatment efficacy, detect virologic failure, and guide timely adjustments to ART regimens.

Comorbidity Management

- **Management of Coinfections**: Integration of care for individuals living with HIV and viral hepatitis, tuberculosis (TB), and non-communicable diseases (e.g., cardiovascular disease, diabetes) to optimize health outcomes.

- **Aging and Long-Term Care**: Addressing age-related comorbidities and chronic conditions among aging populations living with HIV/AIDS through multidisciplinary care and geriatric assessments.

Challenges and Limitations

Drug Resistance and Adverse Effects

- **Antiretroviral Resistance**: Emergence of drug-resistant HIV strains due to incomplete adherence, suboptimal drug levels, and inadequate virologic suppression, necessitating second- and third-line therapies.
- **Long-Term Toxicities**: Potential adverse effects of ART, including metabolic disorders, cardiovascular complications, bone mineral density loss, and renal impairment, requiring monitoring and management.

Access and Equity

- **Global Treatment Disparities**: Disparities in ART access, affordability, and healthcare infrastructure, particularly in low- and middle-income countries (LMICs) and marginalized populations, hindering universal treatment coverage.
- **Stigma and Discrimination**: Societal stigma, discrimination, and legal barriers impacting HIV/AIDS care-seeking behaviors, treatment adherence, and retention in care among affected individuals.

Future Directions and Innovations

Novel Drug Development

- **Next-Generation Antiretrovirals**: Development of novel antiretroviral agents with improved pharmacokinetic profiles, reduced toxicity, and activity against multidrug-resistant HIV strains.
- **Broadly Neutralizing Antibodies (bNAbs)**: Harnessing bNAbs as adjunctive therapies or for HIV prevention

strategies, including long-acting formulations for passive immunization.

Curative Strategies

- **Functional Cure Approaches**: Advancing therapeutic vaccines, latency-reversing agents, and gene editing technologies toward achieving sustained virologic remission or eradication of HIV reservoirs.
- **Gene Therapy and Immunomodulation**: Exploration of gene editing tools (e.g., CRISPR/Cas9) and immune modulation strategies to enhance immune responses against HIV and target viral reservoirs.

Conclusion

Advances in HIV/AIDS treatment strategies have transformed the prognosis and quality of life for individuals living with the virus, shifting from life-threatening illness to manageable chronic condition with long-term adherence to ART. Ongoing research, innovation, and global collaboration are essential to address remaining challenges, including drug resistance, treatment access disparities, and long-term health outcomes. By leveraging scientific advancements, optimizing treatment regimens, and prioritizing patient-centered care, the goal of achieving durable viral suppression, enhancing health equity, and ultimately ending the HIV/AIDS epidemic remains within reach.

Printed in Dunstable, United Kingdom